Molecular Genetics

Other books in the Biomedical Sciences Explained Series

0 7506 32569   Biochemistry *J.C. Blackstock*
0 7506 28790   Biological Foundations *N. Lawes*
0 7506 32542   Biology of Disease *W. Gilmore*
0 7506 31112   Cellular Pathology *D.J. Cook*
0 7506 28782   Clinical Biochemistry *R. Luxton*
0 7506 24574   Haematology *C.J. Pallister*
0 7506 32550   Human Genetics *A. Gardner, R.T. Howell and T. Davies*
0 7506 34138   Immunology *B.M. Hannigan*
0 7506 34154   Transfusion Science *J. Overfield, M. Dawson and D. Hamer*

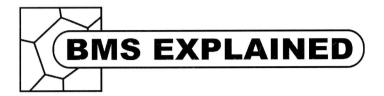

Molecular Genetics

J.T. Hancock BSc PhD
Senior Lecturer in Molecular Cell Biology, University of the West of England, Bristol, UK

Series Editor:
C.J. Pallister PhD MSc FIBMS CBiol MIBiol CHSM
Principal Lecturer in Haematology, Department of Biological and Biomedical Sciences,
University of the West of England, Bristol, UK

BUTTERWORTH HEINEMANN

OXFORD AUCKLAND BOSTON JOHANNESBURG MELBOURNE NEW DELHI

Butterworth-Heinemann
Linacre House, Jordan Hill, Oxford OX2 8DP
225 Wildwood Avenue, Woburn, MA 01801-2041
A division of Reed Educational and Professional Publishing Ltd

℞ A member of the Reed Elsevier plc group

First published 1999

British Library Cataloguing in Publication Data
A catalogue record for this book is available from the British Library

Library of Congress Cataloguing in Publication Data
A catalogue record for this book is available from the Library of Congress

ISBN 0 7506 3253 4

Data manipulation by David Gregson Associates, Beccles, Suffolk
Printed and bound in Great Britain by Bath Press plc, Bath, Avon

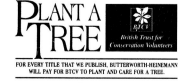

Contents

To Mum, Dad and Peter –
and to Annabel,
who missed out last time
by about two weeks

Preface

Molecular genetics has become an integral part of modern biology and is frequently a topic for discussion in today's media, both newspapers and television. The aim of this book is to give an introduction to the subject suitable for undergraduates studying in the first two years of their degree.

The book is divided into two sections. Part One concentrates on the molecular aspects of genetics, describing the structure of DNA and how it is used by the cellular machinery to encode and synthesize proteins. Part Two concentrates on the methodologies employed by molecular geneticists in the laboratory. Clearly it is not possible here to include all the techniques used in a modern laboratory, or indeed to describe them in enough detail to be used as a recipe book, but a brief explanation of the most common methods is given, illustrated with real results from experiments performed in a working research laboratory.

The last chapter concentrates on the uses and the future of molecular genetics, including a discussion of the biotechnology industry, transgenics and gene therapy. Included here is a very brief discussion of the ethics of such work, and it is hoped that readers may consider these more deeply as they study.

Suggested further reading is given at the end of each chapter, and this is primarily in the form of reviews and other textbooks, rather than primary research papers. However, Chapter 1 is an introductory chapter, and as such many of the excellent genetics textbooks published have been listed here. Although these also cover material found in subsequent chapters, the repetitive listing of these texts has been avoided. Therefore, the reader is guided to the end of Chapter 1 as an excellent place at which to start further reading.

As with all the books in this series, each chapter starts with learning objectives, while ending with key facts and self-assessment questions. It is hoped that readers find these useful.

During the writing of this book, I, like all authors of textbooks, have been supported by many people throughout the project. I would like to thank my colleagues in the Biochemistry and Molecular Biology Group at UWE for the many conversations which have been useful to the content of the book. I am very grateful to Dr Radhika Desikan for supplying the photographs from her research which have helped to illustrate this text. I would like to thank Dr Chris Pallister, who invited me to write the book and subsequently edited it, and also the team at Butterworth-Heinemann for their support and help.

Finally I would like to thank my wife, Sally-Ann, for all her help and support, and Thomas and Annabel for not pressing the delete key at vital moments.

J.T. Hancock

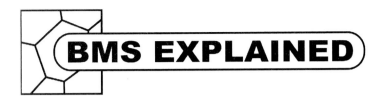

Series preface

The many disciplines that constitute the field of Biomedical Sciences have long provided excitement and challenge both for practitioners and for those who lead their education. This has never been truer than now as we ready ourselves to face the challenges of a new millennium. The exponential growth in biomedical enquiry and knowledge seen in recent years has been mirrored in the education and training of biomedical scientists. The burgeoning of modular BSc (Hons) Biomedical Sciences degrees and the adoption of graduate-only entry by the Institute of Biomedical Sciences and the Council for Professions Supplementary to Medicine have been important drivers of change.

The broad range of subject matter encompassed by the Biomedical Sciences has led to the design of modular BSc (Hons) Biomedical Sciences degrees that facilitate wider undergraduate choice and permit some degree of specialization. There is a much greater emphasis on self-directed learning and understanding of learning outcomes than hitherto.

Against this background, the large, expensive standard texts designed for single subject specialization over the duration of the degree and beyond, are much less useful for the modern student of biomedical sciences. Instead, there is a clear need for a series of short, affordable, introductory texts, which assume little prior knowledge and which are written in an accessible style. The *Biomedical Sciences Explained* series is specifically designed to meet this need.

Each book in the series is designed to meet the needs of a level 1 or 2 student and will have the following distinctive features:

- written by experienced academics in the biomedical sciences in a student-friendly and accessible style, with the trend towards student-centred and life-long learning firmly in mind;
- each chapter opens with a set of defined learning objectives and closes with self-assessment questions which check that the learning objectives have been met;
- aids to understanding such as potted histories of important scientists, descriptions of seminal experiments and background information appear as sideboxes;
- extensively illustrated with line diagrams, charts and tables wherever appropriate;
- use of unnecessary jargon is avoided. New terms are explained, either in the text or sideboxes;
- written in an explanatory rather than a didactic style, emphasizing conceptual understanding rather than rote learning.

I sincerely hope that you find these books as helpful in your studies as they have been designed to be. Good luck and have fun!

C.J. Pallister

Part One
Molecular Biology

Chapter 1

Introduction

Learning objectives

After studying this chapter you should confidently be able to:

Explain the importance of genetics.

Outline the impact genetics is making on modern society.

Appreciate some of the history of genetic discoveries.

Identify the people who made some of the fundamental discoveries in the world of genetics.

Why do we study molecular genetics?

Molecular genetics and the manipulation of an organism's genes have become household concepts in the latter part of the 20th century. We hear about great breakthroughs on the news, and can read about such issues in fiction books and marvel at the images portrayed in the cinema as today's graphics bring the results of fictional genetic manipulation to life. But what does it all mean to us in the everyday world?

Genetics is undoubtedly here to stay, whether we like it or not. It may be that researchers are studying the genetics or altering the genes of organisms as a mere academic exercise, but more and more the results are exerting, or potentially exerting, tangible influences on our lives.

Academics have been puzzled about the functioning of the genetic make-up of organisms, particularly humans, for decades and will no doubt continue to forge ahead with new discoveries, often for what appears to be very little reason to those outside the field. However, the manipulation of genes has helped a great deal in the unravelling of the biochemistry and physiology of organisms. Consider questions such as:

- Where is it likely that a particular protein is being expressed in the body?
- What influences the presence of a protein in tissues?
- How many related types of a protein might be present?

Gene therapy usually allows the placing of a gene within a person in cells which will not influence the next generation. This means transferring the genes to somatic cells, and therefore this is referred to as somatic gene therapy. Germ line gene therapy, where the sex cells are manipulated, is banned.

- And, very importantly, how is that protein functioning at a molecular level?

These and many other questions may all be answered using molecular genetic techniques, and would be much more difficult to answer if genetic techniques were not available. Even these questions may seem academic, unless you consider the question of what has gone wrong with that protein to cause that disease? Here, genetics may potentially have a great impact. Once the disease has been characterized as being the result of a genetic defect, the genetic engineers may strive to find a way of altering the defect and replacing the genetic blueprint of the patient with the correct one, and so offer a longer term and lasting cure. Such technology, referred to as **gene therapy**, has to date not been fruitful, but the results are potentially not far away.

It is not only in the arena of direct medical breakthroughs that the benefits of the advancement of genetic engineering might be seen. The biotechnology and pharmaceutical industries are also being aided greatly by this technology. History has witnessed the introduction of recombinant insulin for human use and hepatitis B virus vaccines rely on the expression of viral surface antigens in yeast. **Protein engineering**, the alteration of native proteins for specific uses, is now being used, amongst other things, to alter the specificity of antibodies, and the phrase 'magic bullet' has been coined to describe antibodies that have been targeted to recognize, for example, tumour cells. Farm animals are now able to function as walking fermenters or **bioreactors**, expressing transgenic proteins for human use, while the disease resistance of plants can be modified. Plants are also being used to produce useful materials such as polymers, and there have been recent reports of 'plastic plants'. Manipulation of the oils made by plants, or even the lipid contents of unicellular organisms, may yield a new fuel which can be used in the face of the world's mineral oil supplies running low.

This growth of molecular biology and its impact on our everyday lives is only just beginning. Recently the news was full of Dolly, the cloned sheep. This was the first time a mammal had been cloned using the genome from an adult cell and Dolly's wool has even been auctioned for charity, highlighting the public awareness of this technology. However, such work has sparked an outcry of protests, and legislation and **ethical committees** are struggling to keep pace with the developments. Already other groups working with mammals are claiming cloning success and, clearly, the future of molecular genetics is an exciting one and one in which we may all be influenced.

A transgenic organism is one in which a new gene or set of genes has been transferred. Often this is used in connection with the placing of genes into the genomes of higher organisms. For example, a sheep which has the gene for a human growth factor and is producing the growth factor in its milk will be referred to as a transgenic sheep. This is discussed further in the final chapter.

A brief history of molecular genetics

Many would agree that genetics started with the plant breeding experiments of **Gregor Mendel**. Before the ideas of Mendel were accepted the characteristics of an organism were thought to be a blending of the traits of the parents, and therefore also influenced by the traits of the grandparents, great-grandparents, etc. Ideas on inheritance were published by **Galton** in 1865 when he wrote two articles on 'Hereditary talent and character', basing his ideas on statistical analysis. In the same year, **Charles Darwin** published *The Origin of Species*, but the actual molecular mechanisms underlying the modes of inheritance and evolution were unknown. Meanwhile, Mendel was embarking on experiments which were to eventually influence the subject of genetics, although at the time his work was virtually ignored. With the breeding of pea plants Mendel obtained the first insights into the inheritance patterns of simple character-istics, and his work was published in 1866 in *Verhandlungen des naturforchenden Vereines* in Brunn. However, although fairly well distributed and read, the scientific community ignored his work until similar experiments were repeated and similar conclusions were drawn by **Hugo De Vries** in the Netherlands, **Carl Correns** in Germany and **Erich von Tschermak** in Austria at the turn of the century.

While Mendel's work stayed in obscurity awaiting rediscovery, in 1869 **Friedrich Miescher** discovered that the nucleus of cells contained DNA, a substance which at the time he named **nuclein**. At about the same time as Mendel's pioneering work was being repeated in 1902, **Archibald Garrod** was studying a disease which is characterized by the presence of a black pigment in the urine, **alkaptonuria**. Garrod was sure that the pigment resulted in the build-up of an intermediate in a biochemical pathway and he noticed that the inheritance pattern of the disease followed that of a Mendelian recessive trait – and, in fact, this was the first genetic disease characterized.

Also in 1902 **Walter Sutton** and **Theodor Boveri** proposed the theory of chromosomes. In 1908 **Godfrey Hardy**, an English mathematician, and **Wilhelm Weinberg**, a German physician, formulated their principle to account for observations made in population genetics. However, one of the greatest breakthroughs in genetics was made by **Thomas Hunt Morgan** with his work on the fruit fly *Drosophila melanogaster* which started in 1910. By studying various traits inherited by this fly, he could demonstrate that the genes resided on chromosomes and could start to map the positions of the genes within the genome. Co-workers in his laboratory included **Calvin Bridges**, **Arthur Sturtevant** and **Hermann Muller**. Much of the work achieved by this group remains fundamental to today's understanding of genetics, with a **genetic map** being published in 1913 and the use of X-rays to induce mutations being reported in 1927.

In 1932 physicists entered the genetics field, notably with a lecture by **Niels Bohr** entitled 'Light and life', presented to an international congress in Copenhagen. Such work led to the

---

Gregor Mendel was born on 22 July 1822 in Heinzendorf, Silesia (now Hyncice) and died 6 January 1884 in Brunn, Austria (now Brno). He was the son of a peasant farmer. He entered the Church in 1843 and joined the Augustinian monastery at Brunn. In 1851 he went to Vienna University where he stayed until 1853. His breeding experiments started in 1856 and he published his results in 1866. He effectively finished his breeding work in 1871, probably because he had become an abbot in 1868 which gave him large amounts of administrative duties.

Thomas Hunt Morgan was born on 25 September 1866 in Hopemont, Kentucky and died 4 December 1945. He attended both Kentucky University and Johns Hopkins University, but in 1903 he moved to Columbia University in New York City, where he did his breeding experiments with the fruit fly *Drosophila melanogaster*. He was awarded the Nobel prize for this work in 1933.

> **Max Delbrück** was born 6 September 1906 in Berlin and died 9 March 1981 in New York. He obtained his PhD from the University of Göttingen in 1930. As one of the founders of the 'Phage Group' he shared the Nobel prize with Luria and Hershey in 1969.

> **James Watson** was born on 6 April 1928 in Chicago while **Francis Crick** was born 8 June 1916 in Northampton. Watson entered University early at the age of 15 and graduated in 1947. He obtained his PhD from the University of Indiana in 1950. Crick obtained his PhD from Cambridge, and it was there that the two met. They were awarded the Nobel prize in 1962.

publication of a book entitled *What is Life?* in 1944 by **Erwin Schrödinger.**

George Beadle and **Edward Tatum** proposed that one gene coded for one enzyme in 1941, a theory that has had to be modified to one gene/one polypeptide based on today's knowledge of genetics. It is now known that certain enzymes are composed of many polypeptides, each requiring their own gene. Beadle and Tatum studied the slime mould *Neurospora*, which they altered by mutagenesis. They then tried to recover lost biochemical activity by the addition of specific intermediates in the biochemical pathways. They were able to show that the defects were the result of alterations in single genes which seemed to follow Mendelian recessive characteristics. Meanwhile, in 1944, **Oswald Avery, Colin Macleod** and **Maclyn McCarty** identified DNA as the true genetic material.

Being influenced by the work of Bohr and Schrödinger, **Max Delbrück** founded the '**Phage Group**' in 1940 – a collection of biologists, chemists and physicists from different laboratories which was to have a major influence on the development of modern molecular genetics.

The structure of the DNA molecule was solved by **James Watson** and **Francis Crick** in 1953 using model building, based on the **X-ray data** from **Rosalind Franklin** and **Maurice Wilkins**. Such information led to the demonstration of the semiconservative nature of DNA replication by **Matthew Meselson** and **Franklin Stahl** in 1958.

Work in the 1960s saw the discovery of messenger RNA in 1961 by **Sidney Brenner, François Jacob** and **Matthew Meselson**, while 1966 saw the genetic code being cracked by **Marshall Nirenberg, Har Gobind Khorana.**

The 1970s saw the first *in vitro* recombinant DNA made by **Paul Berg** and the first use of a plasmid to clone DNA by **Herb Boyer** and **Stanley Cohen**. Such technology is commonplace today. More recent developments which have also reached common status in most laboratories today include the polymerase chain reaction, pioneered by the Cetus Corporation.

Suggested further reading

Brown, T.A. (1998). *Genetics: A Molecular Approach*, 3rd edn. Chapman and Hall. (Highly recommended.)

Hartl, D.L. (1994). *Genetics*, 3rd edn. Jones and Bartlett.

Hartl, D.L. and Jones, E.W. (1999). *Essential Genetics*, 2nd edn. Jones and Bartlett.

Lewin, B. (1997). *Genes VI*. Oxford University Press.

McConkey, E.H. (1993). *Human Genetics: The Molecular Revolution*. Jones and Bartlett.

Mirsky, A.E. (1968). The discovery of DNA. *Scientific American*, **218**, 78–88.

Morgan, T.H. (1910). Sex-limited inheritance in *Drosophila*. *Science*, **32**, 120–122.

Olby, R.C. (1966). *Origins of Mendelism*. Constable.

Peters, J.A. (1959). *Classic Papers in Genetics*. Prentice Hall.

Russell, P.J. (1998). *Genetics*, 5th edn. Longman (AWL).

Sambrook, J., Fritsch, E.F. and Maniatis, T. (1989). *Molecular Cloning: A Laboratory Manual*, 2nd edn. Cold Spring Harbor Laboratory Press.

Shine, I. and Wrobel, S. (1976). *Thomas Hunt Morgan, Pioneer of Genetics*. University Press of Kentucky.

Stryer, L. (1995) *Biochemistry*, 4th edn. Freeman. (Various useful chapters.)

Watson, J.D. and Crick, F.H.C. (1953). Molecular structure of nucleic acids. *Nature*, **171**, 737–738.

Watson, J.D. and Crick, F.H.C. (1953). Genetic implication of the structure of deoxyribonucleic acid. *Nature*, **171**, 964–967.

Watson, J.D., Gilman, M., Witkowski, J. and Zoller, M. (1992). *Recombinant DNA*. Scientific American Books. (An excellent text and a good source of references.)

Weaver, R.F. and Hedrick, P.W. (1991) *Basic Genetics*. Wm. C. Brown Publishers.

Self-assessment questions

1. What name is given to the technology which allows the replacement of a defective gene in a person's genome, thus curing a genetic disease?
2. Who was the person recognized by many as being the father of modern genetics?
3. Who rediscovered Mendel's work by drawing similar conclusions?
4. What was the first genetic disease characterized?
5. Which species did Thomas Hunt Morgan work on?
6. Who first proposed that one gene encoded one enzyme?
7. Why has the hypothesis in the previous question had to be modified?
8. Who solved the structure of DNA?

Key Concepts and Facts

Introduction

- Genetics is now regularly featured in the press and other news media.

- Genetics has a growing impact on today's society.

- Industries based on biotechnology and pharmaceuticals are very interested in modern molecular genetic techniques.

History

- Modern genetics was thought by many to be started by Gregor Mendel.

- Mendel's work was mainly ignored.

- Miescher discovered that the nucleus of cells contained DNA.

- Thomas Hunt Morgan's work was instrumental to early genetics and his group started gene mapping.

- Delbrück founded the Phage Group in 1940.

- DNA structure was solved by Watson and Crick in 1953.

- Matthew Meselson and Franklin Stahl suggested the semi-conservative nature of DNA replication in 1958.

- The genetic code was cracked by Marshall Nirenberg, Har Gobind and Khorana in 1966.

Chapter 2
What is DNA?

Learning objectives

After studying this chapter you should confidently be able to:

Define what the molecular units of DNA are.

Explain how the molecular units of DNA can come together to form a DNA molecule.

Describe the three-dimensional structure of DNA.

Outline some of the techniques which led to the elucidation of the structure of DNA.

Explain how DNA replicates and the processes involved.

The molecular structure of DNA

In the mid-1940s Avery, Macleod and McCarty identified DNA as the molecular material that made up genes, and by the mid-1950s Watson and Crick, using the data from Franklin and Wilkins, had determined the structure of DNA. But what actually is DNA?

DNA is a very large and very long molecule which is used by cells to store the information needed to make proteins. Therefore the structure of this molecule must allow for the storage and retrieval of that information, and on cell division must allow for the information to be copied and passed on to the daughter cells.

The simplest way of looking at the structure of DNA is as two strings of molecular units, almost like beads on a string. These wind around each other in what has been called the double helix, which was, in fact, the title of Watson's book, a work that he wrote after the DNA structure was published. However, the first complication arises when one realizes that the strings of beads have a direction to them, where the ends are different. On closer examination of the double helix structure, we see that the two strings of beads are held together, but in fact run in opposite directions.

Before we consider this structure further we should look at the structure of an individual string of beads or DNA strand. Each strand can be seen to be made of repeating units, the beads.

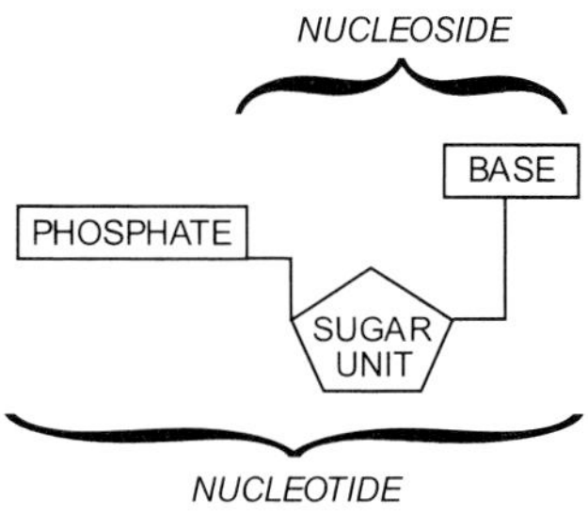

Figure 2.1 *Simplified diagram of the monomer units found in DNA. Here we find a sugar, a base and a phosphate unit joined together to form the basic framework of the DNA molecule*

The joining together of similar units, referred to as monomers, into larger units known as polymers is a common phenomenon in biological systems. The other common examples seen are proteins, where amino acids are joined into long chains called polypeptides.

However, each of these is one of only four types, and each of these types is related and is, in fact, very similar.

Each of the simplified units shown in Figure 2.1 is referred to as a monomer, and many of these will join together, or polymerize, to make the polymer we call DNA. However, this is a simplified diagram and we shall look at each of the components of this monomer separately.

The sugar involved

The sugar found in DNA is a five carbon sugar, otherwise known as a **pentose sugar**. These sugars can exist in two forms, either as a ring structure or as a long, five carbon chain. However, it is the ring form which is found here, as depicted in Figure 2.2. One of the important points to see here is that the $2'$ carbon (pronounced 'two prime carbon') has no OH group attached to it, unlike the $1'$ and $3'$ carbons around the ring, and hence this sugar is called **$2'$-deoxyribose**. In RNA, the $2'$ carbon does attach to an OH group, and here we can see one of the major differences between DNA and RNA.

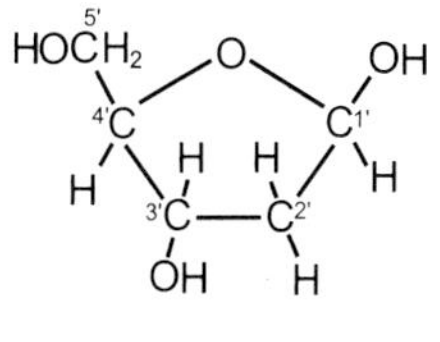

Figure 2.2 *Molecular structure of $2'$-deoxyribose*

The nucleoside

A sugar unit as described above is attached to a second unit known as a **base** or, more correctly, as a nitrogenous base due to its nitrogen atom content. Together, the sugar and the base are collectively called a **nucleoside**. In DNA there are only four types of base, and so four types of monomer units exist. It is also here that the information which is stored in the DNA molecule is found because, as we shall see, it is the order of these bases in the polymer which ultimately determines the protein which is being encoded by a particular stretch of DNA polymer.

Pyrimidines

Thymine

Cytosine

Figure 2.3 *The four bases found in DNA*

Purines

Adenine

Guanine

The four bases can be separated into two groups, each group having two members. The simplest bases are the **pyrimidines**, which have a single ring structure. The two forms found in DNA are thymine and cytosine. The other bases are the **purines**, where there are two rings found in the structure. The forms found in DNA are adenine and guanine. All four structures are shown in Figure 2.3.

The phosphates

To complete the monomer structure requires the addition of a phosphate unit to the nucleoside. Once this happens the whole monomer unit is referred to as a **nucleotide**. In a nucleotide we find three phosphate groups which have been joined in a long chain, as seen in Figure 2.4. Here we should just note that the phosphate groups are labelled α, β and γ.

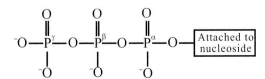

Figure 2.4 *The phosphate chai to complete the nucleotide st·*

Figure 2.5 *Molecular structure of a complete nucleotide. Here, incorporation of cytosine is used as an example*

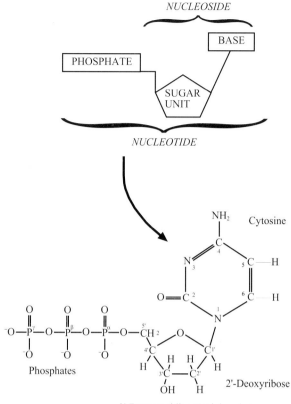

2'-Deoxycytidine 5'-triphosphate

DNA is a polymer of nucleotide units

We can see that the unitary structure of DNA is the nucleotide monomer, made up of a sugar, a phosphate chain and a base, where the base is any one of four. The basic nucleotide is shown in Figure 2.5, where a nucleotide containing the base cytosine is used as an example.

However, as we have a choice of four bases which can be incorporated into the nucleotide, we have four nucleotides which can be used to make DNA. These are:

- 2'-deoxythymidine 5'-triphosphate, using thymine as the base;
- 2'-deoxyguanosine 5'-triphosphate, using guanine as the base;
- 2'-deoxyadenosine 5'-triphosphate, using adenine as the base;
- 2'-deoxycytidine 5'-triphosphate, using cytosine as the base.

Fortunately, these are usually abbreviated to dTTP, dGTP, dATP and dCTP, respectively, where the 'd' denotes that the sugar is the deoxy form, while the first letter refers to the base incorporated. Even more conveniently, short abbreviations are used, that is, T, G, A and C.

Unused phosphate attached to
5' carbon of sugar

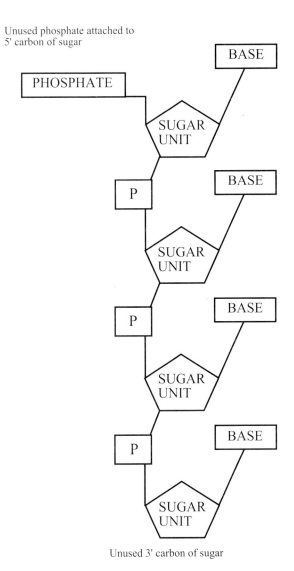

Figure 2.6 *Simplified diagram to show the structure of a polynucleotide*

Unused 3' carbon of sugar

Therefore, we have the building blocks prepared and can now polymerize these to form a long chain, or **polynucleotide**. Here, the nucleotides are held together by the bonding of the 3' carbon of the deoxyribose sugar to the first or α phosphate group of the next nucleotide. This bond is referred to as a **phosphodiester** bond, and results in the β and γ phosphate groups of the bonding phosphate chain being lost. This bis-phosphate by-product is further cleaved to yield inorganic phosphate P_i, with a release of energy. A simplified polynucleotide is shown in Figure 2.6.

Several important points need to be noted:

- As hinted at earlier, the resulting polynucleotide has a direction to it, that is, the ends are not the same. At one end there is still a triphosphate unit attached to the 5' carbon of the sugar, and

As DNA was originally isolated from the nucleus of eukaryotic cells, and because it is an acidic compound, it is referred to as a nucleic acid. Now this term is used to describe polynucleotides in general, and therefore includes RNA.

therefore this end of the chain is called the $5'$ end (pronounced 'five prime'). At the other end is an unused $3'$ ('three prime') carbon still attached to an untouched OH group. This is the $3'$ end of the chain. Further polymerization could still take place but, even if it did, we still end up with a $5'$ end and a $3'$ end.

- The phosphate groups contain a negative charge due to the dissociation of a proton from an OH group, leaving O^-. Therefore the molecule is both acidic and negatively charged, a useful characteristic which we will encounter later in Part Two.

- Most importantly for the function of DNA, as we go down a chain we encounter a series of sugars, all identical, a series of phosphate groups forming phosphodiester bonds, all identical, but also a series of bases and, as any base can be incorporated at any point, then we have a **large amount of variation** in the order of the bases. For example, with our polynucleotide of four bases in Figure 2.6, we could have drawn the bases in the order A-T-C-G, or in the order T-A-C-G, or in the order A-A-T-C, etc. In fact there are $4 \times 4 \times 4 \times 4$ variations, 256 in all, and that is with only four nucleotides. When you then consider that a DNA molecule has a chain length of many thousands of nucleotides, the variation becomes almost infinite.

The three-dimensional structure of DNA

X-ray diffraction

A variety of X-ray sources are available to the modern biochemist. Many laboratories have small, low powered X-ray sources which can be used if the sample has formed particularly good crystals, or to get preliminary data. High powered X-ray sources are available at synchrotron centres such as at Daresbury, UK. Such facilities are expensive to use and often require a long wait for available time.

The structures of many biological molecules, including that of DNA and many proteins, can be elucidated by an experimental method known as **X-ray diffraction**. In this method, the material under study is first crystallized and then held in the path of an X-ray beam. The X-rays falling on the crystal are deflected, or more accurately diffracted, at particular angles, depending on the spacings of the atoms in the molecule. The exact deflection angle and the intensity of the deflected beams are measured by a photographic film which is held in the path of the X-ray beams generated. This gross oversimplification of the method is depicted in Figure 2.7.

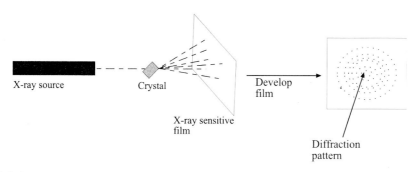

Figure 2.7 *Simplified diagram of X-ray diffraction*

The pattern obtained on the film is known as a **diffraction pattern** and by measuring both the position and the intensity of the spots obtained the researcher can gain a large amount of information about the spacings of the atoms in the molecule. A conversion of the spots into a sensible model and ultimately the whole structure of the molecule requires large amounts of quite complex mathematics, which is well beyond the scope of this book. However, it is exactly this type of approach that led Watson and Crick to the double helix model for DNA.

Base ratio determinations

As well as the X-ray patterns available for the determination of the structure of DNA, another rather interesting piece of information was available. At Columbia University **Erwin Chargaff** was trying to determine the exact composition of the bases within a DNA molecule. The method he used was **paper chromatography**.

The results that were obtained were a crucial hint to the DNA structure. What the experiments showed was that the amount of adenine in any DNA was exactly equal to the amount of thymine, and moreover that the amount of guanine seen was exactly equal to the amount of cytosine. Therefore, the total number of purine bases in a DNA molecule was equal to the number of pyrimidine bases in the molecule.

The double helix

What Watson and Crick realized was that DNA consisted of two polynucleotide strands, which run in opposite directions. Further, these strands were wound around each other to form a double helix. The sugars and phosphate groups effectively form the staging of the helix and make two continuous strands from one end to the other. Sticking out from this staging and, more importantly, pointing inwards, are the bases. These bases are like the steps on a spiral staircase. What Watson and Crick also realized was that the bases come into contact with each other and therefore each step of the staircase is actually two bases, holding each other's 'hands' by way of **hydrogen bonding**.

The interactions seen on the steps of the DNA are shown in Figure 2.8. As can be seen, thymine on one strand always hydrogen bonds to adenine on the other strand while cytosine always hydrogen bonds to guanine. Therefore, once we know the sequence of the bases on one strand we automatically know the sequence of the other strand, because we know that each base has to align with its other counterpart. The two strands are said to be **complementary** to each other, and the phrase 'complement strand' is often used. The second point to notice from Figure 2.8 is that there are three hydrogen bonds between guanine and cytosine, while there are only two hydrogen bonds between adenine and thymine. As the two

Erwin Chargaff obtained his PhD in Vienna in 1928, and by 1950 had made a significant contribution to modern molecular biology. However, he was a vocal critic of the subject. His autobiography, *Heraclitean Fire: Sketches From a Life Before Nature*, was published by Rockefeller University Press, New York, in 1978.

Hydrogen atoms which are attached to one atom can be attracted by the relatively negative charge of another atom. Effectively, the hydrogen atom becomes shared between the two competing atoms and the result is an attraction of two different parts of a molecule, and a bonding is created. Although relatively weak and easy to break, when many hydrogen bonds are involved, as with DNA, it is definitely a case of strength in numbers, and the overall result can be very strong bonding.

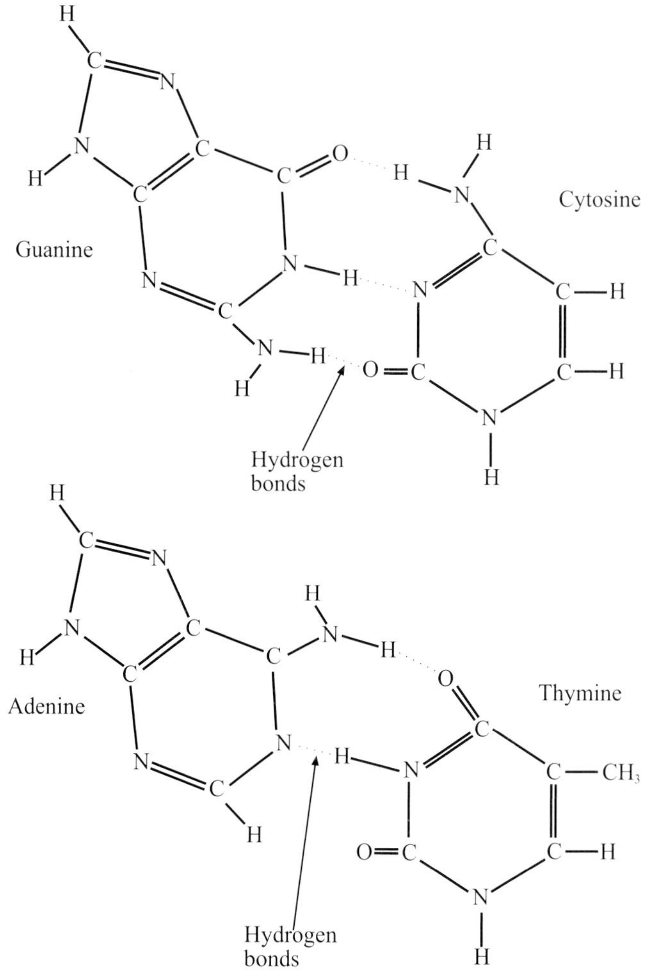

Figure 2.8 *Hydrogen bonding seen between bases in the DNA molecule*

strands of DNA are only held together by these bonds, the total number of bonds between the bases of two strands becomes important when trying to estimate the stability of the molecule. Such matters will be readdressed in Part Two.

If a model is made of the DNA molecule, it becomes apparent that the helix has a regular pattern. The helix is, in fact, approximately 20 Å across, and has two grooves running around and along it. One groove is referred to as the wide groove, while the other is the narrow groove. One total rotation of the molecule takes place every 34 Å along, while the distance between the bases, the step height so to speak, is 3.4 Å. A simplified diagram is shown in Figure 2.9.

Further structure to the DNA molecule

As well as the DNA double helix as described by Watson and Crick and discussed above, further X-ray diffraction studies have revealed

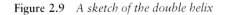

Figure 2.9   *A sketch of the double helix*

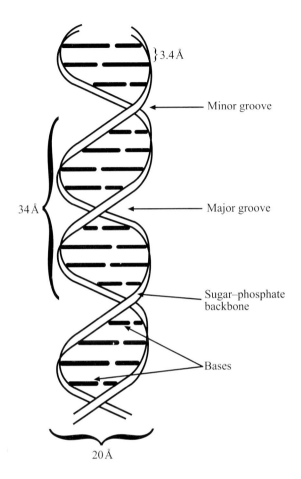

Table 2.1   *Double helical structures identified for DNA*

Form	Direction of helix	Diameter of helix	Bases per turn	Distance between base pairs	Comments
B	Right-handed	19 Å	10	3.4 Å	Watson and Crick model
A	Right-handed	23 Å	11	2.6 Å	
C	Right-handed	19 Å	9.3	3.3 Å	
Z	Left-handed	18 Å	12	3.7 Å	

other double helical structures which DNA may adopt. These are summarized in Table 2.1.

Along with those listed in the table, two other forms, D and E, have also been proposed, although the A and B forms are the favoured naturally occurring ones. However, the most different amongst them is the **Z form**. Here the helix is left-handed! The nucleotide sequence of the DNA appears to be influential in the structure adopted and areas of naturally occurring DNA have been identified which take up the Z form structure. The significance of this is as yet unknown.

The DNA molecule as described is like a long piece of string, but in the cell it has to be packaged neatly and efficiently. One way of achieving this is to wind up the DNA by twisting it into a structure known as a **supercoil**. This can only be achieved if the ends of the DNA are prevented from rotating, for example if the DNA is circular as in a plasmid. Enzymes known as **topoisomerases** can introduce or remove turns in the DNA double helix and, if this is done, the DNA twists up into a helical structure, that is the double helix as described is then further twisted into a helix. This super-coiling may be **positive supercoiling**, resulting from the addition of turns to the double helix, or alternatively **negative supercoiling** as a result of the removal of turns from the helix.

Therefore, we now know molecular structure of a DNA mol-ecule, and such a structure enables us to account for the storage of information as a series of bases in a readable order down the DNA strand. However, the second important feature of DNA that must be accounted for, as well as the coding of proteins, is the fact that it has to replicate. Moreover, this replication has to be completely accurate, to ensure that the information contained in the DNA is not lost or scrambled.

DNA replication

Every cell in a body which synthesizes proteins must contain the appropriate DNA encoding for that information, and if we consider that all the cells are derived from a single cell in the very early stages of development, then DNA has to be replicated many millions of times in order for all the cells to receive their comple-ment.

When approaching the replication of a double-stranded molecule from a logical point of view, there are several ways of obtaining the same objective:

1. The whole molecule could be replicated into a new molecule, where the old DNA remains the same and the new DNA is made of all new components. This would be referred to as **con-servative replication**.
2. The DNA could be broken up and new bits added in a random pattern, so both strands of both resulting DNA molecules contain old and new components. Such a scheme would be **dispersive replication**.
3. We could unzip the DNA into two single strands and use each one of these to form the basis of the new DNA molecules, as depicted in Figure 2.10.

This type of replication is referred to as **semiconservative replica-**

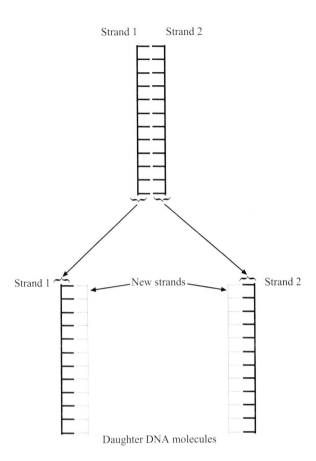

Strand 1   Strand 2

Strand 1   New strands   Strand 2

Daughter DNA molecules

Figure 2.10 *Simple scheme to show semiconservative replication of* DNA

tion and is, in fact, the method used by cells. Using the heavy nitrogen atom ^{15}N to label DNA in *Escherichia coli* cells, allowing their replication and then analysing the results by density gradient centrifugation, in 1957 **Meselson and Stahl** unequivocally identified DNA which was composed of one strand from the old DNA molecule along with a new strand – the result we would expect from semiconservative replication is depicted in Figure 2.10.

But how is such replication achieved? Firstly the DNA is in a double helical structure and therefore, for each of the new DNA molecules to receive an old strand, this helical structure has to be unzipped. Secondly, the new DNA has to be synthesized.

Unwinding of the DNA helix can be carried out by the same group of enzymes as can introduce supercoiling as described above, i.e. **topoisomerases**. These enzymes fall into two groups, Type I and Type II. Type I enzymes have a mechanism whereby they only break one of the DNA strands, while Type II enzymes break both DNA strands. One of the most well-known examples is an enzyme known as **DNA gyrase**.

Once the DNA has been unwound the two strands have to be parted, as depicted in Figure 2.11. This starts at a point known as the **replication origin**. The DNA strands are teased apart by

Figure 2.11 *The start of DNA replication. The DNA strands are parted at an origin of replication, which results in two replication forks. One of the instrumental enzymes here is helicase, aided by SSBs (single-strand binding proteins)*

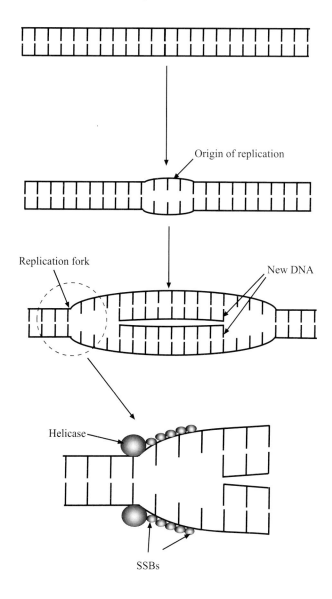

breakage of the hydrogen bonding between the bases, a process which must continue down the strands to enable the replication to proceed. This is catalysed by an enzyme called a **helicase** and the break points are referred to as the replication forks. However, DNA would naturally reanneal back to the double helix with the reformation of the double bonds if allowed to do so. Therefore, proteins known as **single-strand binding proteins** (SSBs) bind to the single-stranded DNA formed by the helicase and stop the reannealing process from taking place.

Once the DNA has been opened up into a single-stranded structure, it is in the position to have the new strand synthesized. However, how does this process start, as the first bases have to be

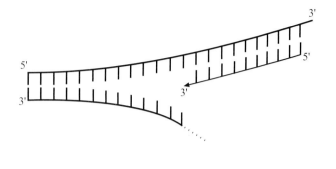

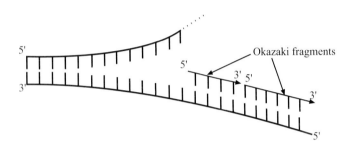

there for strand extension to take place? The process starts by using a **primer**. This is a short length of RNA synthesized by an enzyme called **RNA polymerase**, or **primase**. The RNA primer can vary in length between 6 and 30 bases, and once in place can be used as the start point for DNA synthesis.

The synthesis of the DNA strand is catalysed by an enzyme called **DNA polymerase**. In *E. coli* there are three DNA polymerases, but types I and III seem to be most essential for DNA replication, the function of type II remaining more obscure. Most of the DNA synthesis is carried out by polymerase III, with polymerase I removing the RNA primers and basically tidying up the missing bits, as will be discussed below. In mammalian systems five polymerases have been identified, referred to by the Greek letters α, β, γ, δ, ε.

The polymerases catalyse, more precisely speaking, the formation of new phosphodiester bonds. The newly formed strand will have a 'free' 3′ OH group on the ribose sugar, and to this the α phosphate of the next nucleotide can be attached, with the formation of the phosphodiester bond and the release of the β-γ phosphates as an orthophosphate unit. However, such a process means that the DNA synthesis always takes place in the 5′–3′ direction. This is fine for synthesis along one strand of the DNA molecule, known as the **leading strand**, as continuous synthesis is achieved, as depicted in Figure 2.12.

However, as the other strand, or **lagging strand**, is being effectively unteased backwards, synthesis along the second strand

Reiji Okazaki used DNA of the bacteriophage T4 as his model system for studying DNA replication. To show the presence of short fragments during replication he studied the incorporation of tritium-labelled thymidine. Pulses of label as short as 2 seconds were used and the fragments obtained analysed by ultracentrifugation.

cannot follow the direction of the replication fork. Therefore, on the second strand the synthesis of the new DNA is discontinuous, a process confirmed by the work of **Okazaki** in 1968. Hence the short stretches of DNA are known as **Okazaki fragments** (see Figure 2.12). Each fragment has to be started by its own RNA primer and so, along this strand, you would find short DNA stretches following short RNA stretches and gaps between. Clearly, this is not acceptable and therefore here the action of polymerase I is crucial. This enzyme removes the RNA nucleotides and continues the DNA synthesis to fill the gaps. The final covalent bonding which joins all the resulting Okazaki fragments together is carried out by an enzyme called **DNA ligase**. We will come across this enzyme again in Part Two as it is fundamental to much DNA manipulation work carried out in laboratories.

Suggested further reading

Avery, O.T.C., Macleod, M. and McCarty, M. (1944). Studies on the chemical nature of the substances inducing transformation of pneumococcal types. *Journal of Experimental Medicine*, **79**, 137–158.

Dickerson, R.E. (1992). DNA structures from A to Z. *Methods in Enzymology*, **211**, 67–111.

Dickerson, R.E., Drew, H.R., Conner, B.N. *et al.* (1982). The anatomy of A-, B- and Z-DNA. *Science*, **216**, 475–485.

Meselson, M. and Stahl, F. (1958). The replication of DNA in *Escherichia coli*. *Proceedings of the National Academy of Sciences, USA*, **44**, 671–682.

Okazaki, T. and Okazaki, R. (1969). Mechanisms of DNA chain growth. *Proceedings of the National Academy of Sciences, USA*, **64**, 1242–1248.

Radman, M. and Wagner, R. (1988). The high fidelity of DNA duplication. *Scientific American*, **259**, 24–30.

Watson, J.D. (1968). *The Double Helix*. Atheneum.

Watson, J.D. and Crick, F.H.C. (1953). Molecular structure of nucleic acids. *Nature*, **171**, 737–738.

Self-assessment questions

1. Why is the **pentose** sugar found in nucleic acids so named?
2. How do the pentose sugars differ in DNA compared to RNA?
3. What is the basic structure of a nucleoside?
4. Which of the bases are classed as pyrimidines and which as purines?
5. How does a nucleotide differ from a nucleoside?
6. Why does a DNA polynucleotide have different ends?
7. Name a technique used to elucidate the structure of DNA, and for which other type of biological molecule is this technique regularly used in an attempt to solve its structure?
8. What holds the strands of DNA together?

9. Why do we know the sequence of a complementary strand of DNA if we know the sequence of the first strand?
10. Name four forms of the DNA helix?
11. Name the enzyme which catalyses the synthesis of new DNA?
12. In which direction does DNA synthesis always take place?

Key Concepts and Facts

Molecular Structure
- DNA is a polymer of repeating units.

- DNA strands run in opposite directions.

- The sugar found in DNA is a pentose sugar: $2'$-deoxyribose.

- A sugar joined to a base is known as a nucleoside.

- DNA contains four bases: adenine (A), guanine (G), thymine (T) and cytosine (C).

- The bases are classed into two groups depending on their structure: pyrimidines or purines.

- Nucleotides bind together to form a polynucleotide; a long chain.

- Bases in the chain can be in any order, giving almost infinite variation.

Three-Dimensional Structure
- X-ray diffraction has been a key technique in the elucidation of DNA structure.

- Base composition was also crucial in elucidating DNA structure.

- DNA is, in fact, two polynucleotide strands running in opposite directions.

- Strands of DNA are held together by hydrogen bonds.

- The sequence of bases on one strand automatically gives us the sequence of bases on the second strand.

- DNA may form several different types of helices, although some are more favoured than others in nature.

Replication
- DNA replication is semiconservative.

- Replication starts at a replication origin.

- The direction of replication is always $5'$–$3'$.

- Continuous replication takes place on the leading strand but synthesis on the lagging strand leads to Okazaki fragments.

Chapter 3
Genes

Learning objectives

After studying this chapter you should confidently be able to:

Define what constitutes a gene.

Describe the structure of a typical gene.

Outline the arrangement of related genes in a genome.

Describe gene duplication.

What are genes?

It has been discussed in the preceding chapters that the genetic information needed to code for the proteins which are required by the cell is stored as a sequence of bases on the DNA. However, there has to be an organization to this information, enabling it to be easily found and retrieved. Therefore, the genetic information is stored in packages, or **genes**, where one gene holds the information for the production of one polypeptide sequence. This idea was first hypothesized by Beadle and Tatum in 1941. As the information is in the form of a series of bases along the DNA molecule, a gene is simply a stretch of DNA, with a defined start site and a defined end (Figure 3.1). It can then be processed as a unit and the information passed on to the machinery which will make the protein.

Interestingly, not all the DNA in a cell may be used for the storage of information, and therefore not all the DNA is used as part of a gene. In humans, over 70% of the DNA is not used in encoding protein sequences. Stretches of DNA that lie between genes are known as **intergenic DNA** (Figure 3.2). Secondly, any stretch of DNA has two strands and therefore the capacity for holding two different sequences of bases, depending on which strand is read. However, a gene will only use the information held by one of the strands, and therefore this has to be borne in

A gene

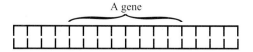

Figure 3.1 *A gene is simply a stretch of DNA*

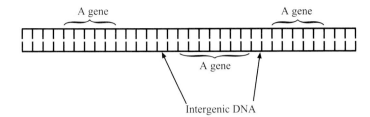

A gene

A gene

A gene

Intergenic DNA

Figure 3.2 *Genes may be on either strand of the DNA molecule*

mind when the information is decoded by both cell and researcher. That is not to say though that both strands are not used. Some genes will be on one strand while others will be of the other strand. Several terms have been coined to refer to the strands which hold the important sequence information and those which do not, such as '**sense**' and '**antisense**', '**coding**' and '**non-coding**', but as T.A. Brown points out in his textbook (*Genetics: A Molecular Approach*), such terms can easily lead to confusion.

As we saw with DNA replication in Chapter 2, the reading of the DNA sequence has a direction to it. Here, a gene sequence is always read from the 3′ end to the 5′ end, and therefore genes which reside on different strands are read in opposite directions; again a fact that needs considering when a researcher is trying to decipher the gene sequence.

> It should be noted that when a gene sequence is written down, it is usually the complementary strand in the 5′ to 3′ direction which is shown, although transcription takes place in the 3′ to 5′ direction along a gene. The complementary strand sequence shown is equivalent to the sequence of the RNA produced by transcription, and is therefore used to translate the nucleotide sequence into the amino acid sequence.

The arrangement of genes

In higher organisms, each cell may contain more than one DNA molecule and these together are known as chromosomes. Usually the DNA is packaged and each DNA molecule may carry thousands of genes. This will be discussed further in Chapter 4.

Along the length of each DNA molecule will be found thousands of genes, and although the spacing of the genes is usually apparently random, often genes may be grouped into clusters of related genes. In bacteria, it is not unusual to have the need to express several genes which are not the same but are related, in that the proteins which are encoded by the genes are required along a common metabolic pathway. Therefore, as all the genes or, more correctly, their encoded products, are needed more or less simultaneously by the cell, it makes sense for the cell to have all such genes together and have a mechanism to express them together. These clusters of genes are known as **operons**.

Probably the most studied operon is known as the lactose operon in *E. coli*. This operon contains three genes which are required for the utilization of lactose as a metabolic fuel in the cell. The operon encodes for a permease to allow entry of the lactose into the cell along with a transacetylase and β-galactosidase used in the

> Humans cells contain 23 pairs of chromosomes and on these there are probably as many as 100 000 genes. However, such numbers are very variable between organisms. *E. coli* only has one chromosome and less than 3000 genes.

When the sequences of the bases of two genes are very similar they are said to be **homologous**. Usually the homology of two gene sequences are expressed as a percentage, with 100% indicating identity. Homology can be easily quantified by computers and many programs are now available, especially via the Internet (see Chapter 13).

metabolic pathway using lactose. The operon also contains all the control sequences needed to ensure efficient expression of the genes together, as further discussed in Chapter 7.

Operons, as briefly outlined above, do not occur in higher organisms, but we still see clusters of genes. Usually we have clusters of genes which either encode for the same protein or very similar proteins. Such sequences are said to be **homologous** as their nucleotide sequences are very similar. Clusters of similar genes are called **multigene families**, and such families roughly fall into two groups. Simple multigene families are clusters of identical or extremely homologous genes, an example being the genes for 5S rRNA. This is a useful feature for genes from which a large amount of product needs to be synthesized very quickly – the processing of a single copy of the gene being inadequate for the demand. In humans, there may be up to two thousand copies of the 5S rRNA gene.

Alternatively, multigene families may be made up of related but different genes. Such an example is the clusters of **globin genes** found in higher organisms. Here, two clusters are found, one for the α-like subunits of haemoglobin and one for the β-like subunits. The β cluster, located on chromosome 11 in humans, contains six globin genes, referred to as ε, $^{G}\gamma$, $^{A}\gamma$, $\Psi\beta_1$, δ and β. Different genes from the cluster are expressed at different times during the development of the animal. $^{G}\gamma$ and $^{A}\gamma$ are expressed during the foetal phase of the development while ε is expressed in the embryonic phase. δ and β are the adult forms. Similarly, the α cluster, on chromosome 16 in humans, contains seven globin genes, three of which are expressed. Again, these genes are expressed differentially during development, the ζ form being an embryonic one and α_1 and α_2 being the adult forms.

Genes clusters come about because of **gene duplication** events in the DNA (Figure 3.3). Firstly, the DNA may contain a single copy of the gene, but this can be duplicated, and therefore the DNA will have two copies of the gene, as depicted in Figure 3.3.

Next, base changes within one or indeed both genes may take place, which means that over time the genes become different, but share similarity where changes have not taken place. Also, there are areas within the base sequence of any one gene that may not be very important, as regions within the protein encoded by that gene may be fairly redundant, and these can be changed without major changes to the protein's function. Therefore, nucleotide changes may take place which do alter the protein sequence quite markedly, but the areas of importance within the protein remain the same, as alterations here would be catastrophic. Such unaltered sequences are often looked for by researchers in related genes as it highlights the areas of importance in proteins and can be used quite often to identify the function of a protein before any function has been assigned through experimentation.

(a) A single copy of the original gene

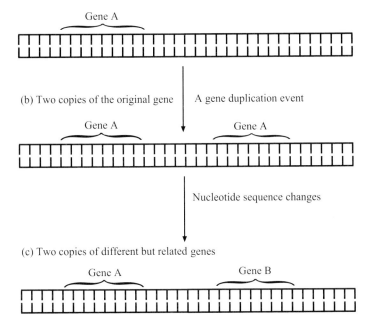

Figure 3.3 *Gene duplication can account for the presence of gene clusters*

Gene A

(b) Two copies of the original gene │ A gene duplication event

Gene A   Gene A

Nucleotide sequence changes

(c) Two copies of different but related genes

Gene A   Gene B

Pseudogenes

Not all genes that can be identified on a chromosome are functional. This is illustrated by the globin cluster of genes. In the β globin cluster there is a gene labelled $\Psi\beta_1$ which, although it appears to be a gene, holds information that is scrambled and does not encode a functional protein. Such genes are referred to as **pseudogenes**. Again, they arise though gene duplication events, but here alterations in the nucleotide sequence are too pronounced to leave the gene usable. The α globin gene cluster contains three such genes.

Genes may not be continuous

Although a gene is a sequences of bases along a length of DNA, this sequence is not necessarily continuous, but rather can be interrupted by non-coding regions. Such a gene is depicted in Figure 3.4.

The stretches of coding DNA are known as **exons**, while the stretches interrupting the coding area are known as **intervening**

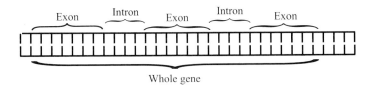

Exon   Intron   Exon   Intron   Exon

Whole gene

Figure 3.4 *Genes may contain introns which do not encode protein sequences*

sequences (IVSs) or (much more commonly) as **introns**. A gene may have no introns or several. For example, the cystic fibrosis transmembrane regulator gene has 26 introns. The mouse β globin gene has approximately half of the gene as introns, and this sort of statistic is not uncommon.

It is important, as far as the cell is concerned, that when the DNA sequence is uncoded, the intron areas have to be ignored. We shall see that the introns are, in fact, transcribed into RNA as the process of gene expression takes place, but later in the process the introns are removed or spliced. This process has to be achieved with great accuracy, firstly to ensure that no coding information is lost, and secondly to ensure that no non-coding information is left in. Therefore there must be features of the introns which are recognized to guide this splicing event.

A simplified rule is that the sequence GT is found at the start of the intron with AG at the end of the intron, giving the gene sequence:

exon/GT-intron-AG/exon

However, four nucleotides seem hardly sufficient to ensure that such an important event takes place properly, and by the use of the technique known as **site-directed mutagenesis**, that is where individual bases are changed in a sequence and the effects studied, **consensus sequences** for the splice sites in genes have been identified. These are shown in Figure 3.5.

The importance of many of these bases in the consensus sequence has been further shown by studying natural mutations, where the splicing of a gene's introns is defective and therefore a non-functioning product is formed. Such mutations have, for example, been found to be responsible for thalassaemia.

The actual process of splicing involves other RNA molecules, called **U-RNA**, or **small nuclear RNAs** (snRNAs). It is a complex process and it must be emphasized that it is one which must be accurate to ensure that no bases are lost or added to the final RNA product.

> Consensus sequences are sequences which are most likely to occur in related genes. Usually such sequences are found by the alignment of several related sequences, and the most likely nucleotides at each position would be quoted in the consensus sequence. Often such sequences contain positions denoted by apparently strange letters; for example, N represents any nucleotide, while Y might represent any pyrimidine. A consensus may be GTNNTYC for example.

Figure 3.5 *The consensus sequences either side of a gene intron. N denotes any nucleotide, while Y denotes either pyrimidine (U or C), R denotes either purine (G or A), and S denotes either A or C*

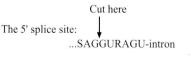

Cut here

The 5' splice site: ...SAGGURAGU-intron

Cut here

The 3' splice site: intron-YYYYYYYYYYYYYYNYAGG...

Suggested further reading

Crick, F.H.C. (1979). Split genes and RNA splicing. *Science*, **204**, 264.

Gilbert, W. (1978). Why genes in pieces? *Nature*, **271**, 501.

Gilbert, W. (1985). Genes in pieces revisited. *Science*, **228**, 823–824.

Padgett, R.A, Grabowski, P.J., Konarska, M.M. and Sharp, P.A. (1985). Splicing messenger RNA precursors: branch sites and lariat RNAs. *Trends in Biochemical Sciences*, **10**, 154–157.

Self-assessment questions

1. Does all the DNA in a genome always encode useful information?
2. In which direction is a gene sequence read?
3. What is an operon?
4. What is a pseudogene?
5. What are the non-coding areas within a gene called?
6. What is a consensus sequence?

Key Concepts and Facts

Genes
- A gene is a stretch of DNA, with a defined start site and a defined end point.

- Genes may be on either strand of the DNA.

- Gene sequences are always read in the 3' to 5' direction.

Arrangements of Genes
- Genes with products which are related, perhaps encoding parts of the same metabolic pathway, may be clustered together in some species.

- Sequences which are related, having similar base sequences, are referred to as homologous.

- Gene duplication may lead to similar and related genes, but ones which have sequence differences due to subsequent mutations.

Genes May Not be Continuous
- The coding parts of a gene are called exons.

- The sequences between the exons are called introns.

- The border sequences of introns allow for their efficient removal during gene expression.

Chapter 4

Genome structure

Learning objectives

After studying this chapter you should confidently be able to:

Outline the structure and life cycle of bacteriophages.

Describe the genomes of eukaryotic specific viruses.

Outline genomes of bacteria, including plasmids.

Define areas of mobile DNA: transposons.

Outline the genomes of eukaryotes.

Describe the structure of chromosomes.

Define extra-nuclear genomes and explain their importance.

The majority of organisms retain their genetic information in the form of DNA, from some of the most simple viruses to the most complex mammals. However, many of these organisms contain large amounts of genetic information, the entire complement of the organism being referred to as its **genome**. Here we will discuss the genomes of many different forms of organisms, as many of the viruses, bacteria and even eukaryotic cells are used as either model systems or experimental tools in today's molecular genetics laboratories.

Bacteriophages

Bacteriophages, or commonly just **phages**, are viruses which attack and use bacteria as host cells. They are composed very simply of only two components:

- A protein coat or **capsid**.
- A nucleic acid, either DNA or RNA.

The protein coats of phages are arranged in one of three basic forms:

1. The **icosahedral form** has the nucleic acid simply surrounded by a three-dimensional pattern of protein subunits, or **protomers**.

An example of this simple form of bacteriophage is the MS2 phage which uses *E. coli* as a host.

2. A second coat structure involves the protein subunits being arranged in a rod formation with the nucleic acid running down through the middle. Such phages are referred to as helical or **filamentous phages**, an example being the M13 phage which again uses *E. coli* as a host.

3. The phages with the most complex structure, however, are known as the **head-and-tail type**. These phages, as depicted in Figure 4.1, have a head structure which resembles an icosahedral virus, on top of a filamentous tail structure, to which is attached a base structure which will be used in host recognition and for entry of the nucleic acid into the host cell. Examples of such viruses are T2, T4, T7 and λ which attack *E. coli*, and SPO1 which uses *Bacillus subtilis* as a host.

The genomes of the phages are very varied. They range from single-stranded RNA or double-stranded RNA to single-stranded circular DNA and double-stranded linear DNA. They are also very varied in size. The MS2 virus mentioned above has a genome size of only 3.6 thousand bases (3.6 kb) containing only three genes. However, the T2 and T4 virus genomes are approximately 166 thousand bases (166 kb) with over 150 genes.

Bacteriophages are commonly used as vehicles, or **vectors**, for the entry of genes into cells and, as such, a brief mention of their life cycle and how they are visualized in the laboratory will be given here. Their life cycle falls into two categories: **lytic** and **lysogenic**.

In the lytic cycle, the bacteriophage recognizes and attaches itself to the host surface, followed by injection of the nucleic acid material into the host. Following this is a latent period, during which new bacteriophage components are manufactured by the host cell. After

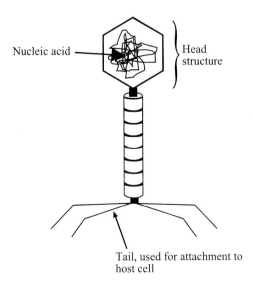

Nucleic acid

Head structure

Tail, used for attachment to host cell

Figure 4.1 *Schematic representation of a typical head-and-tail bacteriophage*

Figure 4.2 *Visualization of phage on an agar plate. Each 'hole' in the bacterial lawn represents the original presence of one phage*

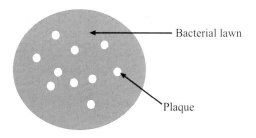

approximately 20 minutes, the host cell bursts and new phages are released which can then go on to infect new cells with the synthesis of yet more phages. Phages which commonly follow the lytic pathway include the T2 and T4 *E. coli* phages. However, in the lysogenic cycle, the phage genome becomes integrated into the genome of the host cell. The phage is now referred to as a **prophage**, while the infected cell is referred to as a **lysogen**. Integration of the phage genes into the host genome takes place through a **recombination event**, as discussed further in Chapter 9, and transcription and expression of the phage genome may be prevented by the production from the phage genome of a **repressor protein**, such as *c*I. The lysogenic state can be maintained for many generations of the host, the genome of the phage being replicated along with that of the host. However, both physical and chemical stimuli may break the lysogenic state and the phage may enter a lytic cycle, with the concomitant synthesis and release of new phages.

To visualize phages in the laboratory, a mixture of bacteria and phages are grown on a solid agar medium. The plate is incubated until the bacteria have formed a **lawn** over the agar surface. However, the presence of phages will mean that bacteria have been lysed and new phages released, which will infect surrounding bacteria and again bacterial lysis will result. After incubation, therefore, one would see a lawn of bacteria which have gaps or **plaques**, with each plaque representing the original presence of a phage. Such a plate can be seen sketched in Figure 4.2.

Viruses that have eukaryotic hosts

Viruses that attack and use eukaryotic cells as hosts are similar in many ways to the phages. However, the basic structures here fall into two classes:

- icosahedral
- filamentous.

Again the genomes of such viruses can be very varied, from single-stranded linear RNA or DNA to double-stranded linear or circular DNA. Also once again, the genome sizes are very varied. Small viruses may have a total genome size of less than 2 kb, containing only four or five genes, while larger genomes are found which contain over 200 genes; for example, the vaccinia virus which uses a mammalian host has a genome size of 240 kb and has 240 genes.

Most of the eukaryotic-specific viruses follow a lytic-type life cycle, but some follow a life cycle more similar to the lysogenic cycle of the phages. Lysogenic cycles may lead to transformation of the host cells, where loss of control of proliferation takes place. With the use of selected viruses in the laboratory, eukaryotic cells may be immortalized, where the loss of the proliferation control means that they will proliferate indefinitely, allowing the researcher to have a constant supply of eukaryotic cells. A typical example here is the use of the Epstein–Barr virus (EBV) to immortalize mammalian lymphocytes. Such techniques have allowed the continued growth and analysis of lymphocytes from patients with certain diseases, such as **chronic granulomatous disease** (CGD).

Chronic granulomatous disease is seen as a lack of the production of free radicals by white blood cells, which means that the patient has an impaired defence against certain pathogens. Usually such patients have recurring infections, but once diagnosed they are prescribed long-term antibiotics.

Retroviruses

Retroviruses are worth singling out because they are RNA-containing viruses and because they encode an enzyme called reverse transcriptase. The RNA molecules contained within retroviruses are single-stranded and between 6 kb and 9 kb long. The genome contains three genes needed for integration of the viral genome into the host genome. These are (see Figure 4.3):

- *gag* – encodes capsid proteins.
- *pol* – encodes proteins needed for viral replication.
- *env* – encodes membrane envelope proteins.

On entry into the cell the RNA has to be copied into DNA which is carried out by the enzyme reverse transcriptase, encoded by *pol*. Once in the form of double-stranded DNA, incorporation into the host genome is possible. This incorporation is random, which may cause problems if such a virus is being used as a gene vector. However, once incorporated, the genes from the virus genome can be expressed and new viruses synthesized.

Reverse transcriptase as an enzyme has been extensively used in molecular genetics. Many researchers study the presence of mRNA in cells as a measure of gene expression. However, RNA is inherently very unstable, and therefore a DNA copy can be made which is much more stable using reverse transcriptase. Such methodology is commonly combined with **polymerase**

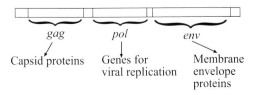

Figure 4.3 *The genes encoded by a typical retrovirus*

Oncogenes are genes which are able to cause a cell to transform, and therefore lead to uncontrolled proliferation of cells and in tissues lead to cancer. The first oncogenes were isolated from retroviruses.

chain reaction (PCR) in a technique referred to as RT-PCR (reverse transcriptase-PCR). This will be discussed further in Chapter 12.

Other research concentrates on retroviruses because the **HIV viruses** which cause the immunodeficiency disease AIDS are retroviruses and because some retroviruses encode **oncogenes**, and therefore may lead to cancer.

Bacterial genomes

The general distinction between prokaryotes and eukaryotes is based on the presence of a nucleus in eukaryotes which contains the genetic material of the cell. In prokaryotes, such a nucleus is missing. However, in many bacteria, detailed studies still reveal a central part of the cell which can be distinguished from the rest, an area known as the **nucleoid**. It is here that the majority of the DNA resides. In *E. coli* for example, the nucleoid contains a single double-stranded circular piece of DNA. However, this piece of DNA is very large, having a molecular weight of approximately 2.8×10^9, with 4.2×10^6 base pairs and a length of 1.4 mm. To accommodate such a relatively large molecule inside the cell, the DNA is supercoiled, as discussed in Chapter 2. Packaging of the DNA also requires the assistance of proteins, some of which resemble the histone family of proteins, as will be discussed later.

Prokaryotes show a great diversity when it come to the size of their genomes. Some cells have relatively small DNA molecules, with perhaps around 10^6 base pairs, while *Salmonella typhimurium* has a genome ten times bigger.

Plasmids

The DNA associated with the nucleoid is not the only DNA contained within bacteria. Small circular DNA also exists. These DNA molecules have an independent existence within the cell, and also carry genes. Such DNA molecules are known as **plasmids**. However, the genes carried by such DNA are usually not encoded by the nucleoid DNA and, furthermore, the genes of plasmids usually encode additional characteristics. For example, plasmids might carry genes which confer antibiotic resistance to the cell.

Plasmids usually contain one area of DNA which acts as an origin of replication and this therefore confers on the plasmid the characteristic of independence, allowing them to multiply within the cell. However, some plasmids may integrate with the main bacterial genome, and in this state are referred to as **episomes**.

Plasmids, too, vary greatly in size. Small ones may only be approximately 1 kb, while very large ones may exceed 250 kb. Individual plasmids are not restricted to single species of bacteria either. While some plasmids are found in a very restricted number of closely related species, others may have wide host specificity. Furthermore, some plasmids exist in large numbers in one particular individual cell. The number of a given plasmid in a cell is known as the **copy number**. If a plasmid has a low copy number it is referred to as being **stringent**, while plasmids with a high copy number are known as **relaxed**. Lastly here, certain plasmids can not co-exist in the same individual cell. They are referred to as being **incompatible**.

Plasmids are of particular interest to the modern molecular geneticist. Genes are commonly inserted into plasmids to enable them to be placed in cells – the basis of much cloning. If the 'new' genes are to be expressed in the cell, considerations like copy number become much more important, as the higher the copy number, the more likely that the protein product will be made in high quantities in the cell. This is obviously important to the biotechnologist who may be trying to produce and sell a product.

Transposons

Genomes of bacteria are not static, but may have quite large changes taking place. This is because of sections of DNA that have the capacity to move around. Such pieces of DNA are called **transposons**. Transposons exist in different forms, the first to be discovered being the **insertion sequences** (IS). These are lengths of DNA that can be inserted into a target gene within the genome. For example, DNA may be able to move from the main DNA molecule of bacteria to be inserted into a plasmid.

Usually such insertion sequences have at either end a short length of DNA known as an **inverted repeat**, i.e. this small length of DNA has the same sequence if read in either direction along the $5'$–$3'$ strand. Between these inverted repeats is a gene which codes for an enzyme, **transposase**, which catalyses the transposition event.

Composite transposons are very similar except that they contain two insertion sequences which flank a length of DNA (see Figure 4.4).

Tn3 transposons are slightly more complicated. This class of transposon is not flanked by insertion sequences but is still able to move around because the transposon contains a gene coding for transposase (Figure 4.4).

Genomes of eukaryotes

Eukaryotes are distinct from prokaryotes in that they have a nucleus and it is here that the vast majority of the genetic information is held. However, many other differences are seen between prokaryotes and eukaryotes. In the latter, the DNA is partitioned, each nucleus containing several DNA molecules, each of which helps to make up a **chromosome**. The DNA is linear in all

The first transposons to be discovered were the insertion sequences, in 1961. Their discovery came from the study of a series of mutations known as the polar mutations which were unusual in that they affected genes in two parts of the genome.

Figure 4.4 *The classes of transposons*

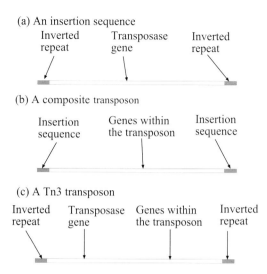

(a) An insertion sequence

Inverted repeat   Transposase gene   Inverted repeat

(b) A composite transposon

Insertion sequence   Genes within the transposon   Insertion sequence

(c) A Tn3 transposon

Inverted repeat   Transposase gene   Genes within the transposon   Inverted repeat

eukaryote nuclei, and in most nuclei there are two copies of each gene. This situation is referred to as the **diploid** complement, while certain cells, for example the sex cells of an individual, will contain only one copy of each gene and are therefore called **haploid**. Lastly, not all the DNA in eukaryotes is contained within the nucleus. Other organelles within the cells, such as mitochondria and chloroplasts, also contain their own complement of functional DNA.

As already seen with viruses and bacteria, here too there is a great variety of genome size. Small genomes in eukaryotes may only be 10–20 thousand kb, while the largest may be 120 million kb. Chromosome number is also very varied. Fruit flies have a haploid chromosome number of only 4 while humans have 23. However, it has become apparent that vast amounts of many eukaryotic genomes are redundant, i.e. not encoding gene products. For the human genome it has been estimated that only 2–3% is actually coding DNA. Of course, if **mutations** take place in the rest, it might mean that there is little or no consequence.

It has been mentioned that DNA in eukaryotes is packaged as chromosomes, but what are they? A chromosome is composed of a length of DNA which is in association with proteins. One of the most important families of protein here is the **histones**. These are very basic proteins, having a relatively high content of the amino acids lysine, arginine and histidine, and they are very conserved in their sequence between different species. To date, there are five histones that have been characterized: H1, H2A, H2B, H3 and H4. They vary in molecular mass from approximately 11 kilodaltons (H4) to 23 kilodaltons (H1).

The DNA and histones are wound up into a complex structure known as the **nucleosome**, and then nucleosomes are associated together, along with the DNA of course, into a chromatin fibre.

One of the most important parts of the chromosome is the **centromere**. This is the point along the chromosome where it is joined to its daughter chromosome in replication, and it is also the point of attachment of the **microtubules** which draw the chromosomes apart so that they can be placed in the new daughter nuclei. The centromere exists along the DNA where there is a special DNA sequence. This sequence is approximately 125 bases long in *Saccharomyces cerevisiae*, while in humans there is a repeating sequence called the **alpha DNA**. In both cases, special proteins also associate with the DNA to form a structure known as the **kinetochore**, and it is to this that the microtubule attaches.

The position of the centromere in different chromosomes is different, as illustrated in Figure 4.5. If the centromere is in the centre of the chromosome it is called **metacentric**, if it is close to one end it is **telocentric**, and if it is inclined to be nearer to one end than the other it is referred to as being **acrocentric**. It is the position of the centromeres in chromosomes which helps researchers to pair up the copies of chromosomes in diploid cells, and such analysis may be useful in identifying individuals who contain too many chromosomes, as in **Down's syndrome** where the patient has an extra chromosome 21, or **Klinefelter's syndrome** where individuals have an extra X sex chromosome (being XXY instead of XY), or when a chromosome is missing, as in **Turner's syndrome** where an individual has a sex chromosome missing and therefore is referred to as being XO.

The ends of chromosomes are known as the **telomeres**. The functions of such areas appear to include the protection of the ends of the DNA, the prevention of DNA joining, and aiding in the replication of DNA. Once again, the DNA has a special sequence

> Down's syndrome occurs at a frequency of approximately 1 in 700, but the chances increase dramatically with the age of the mother. Turner's syndrome, which leads to the affected females being sterile, is less common (1 in 5000).

(a) Metacentric

(b) Submetacentric

(c) Acrocentric

(d) Telocentric

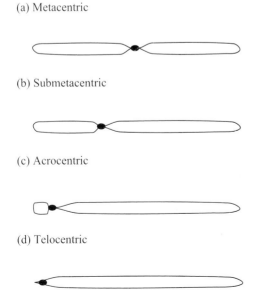

Figure 4.5 *The positions of centromeres on chromosomes*

associated with it here, in this case the multiple repeating of a short sequence, and the telomere also has association with special proteins not found elsewhere in the chromosome. Telomeres have recently come to prominence in the press because their length is thought to change with age, and it has been suggested that regulation of the telomere length might allow cells to survive longer.

DNA outside the nucleus

Certain cellular organelles contain their own genomes which are not only active but also vital to cellular function. Expression of the genes of such organelles is interesting as it will be seen that many of the proteins encoded here are parts of large and important protein complexes, the other polypeptides in the complexes being encoded by the nuclear genome.

Mitochondria

Mitochondria contain a circular piece of DNA which is functionally active. In many mitochondria there is more than one copy of this molecule, for example in humans each mitochondrion probably has ten copies. The size of mitochondrial genomes though is greatly varied. The human mitochondrial DNA is just over 16.5 kb long, while in some plants it is considerably larger. For example, members of the brassica family have a mitochondrial genome of 218 kb while some plants have been reported with mitochondrial genomes over ten times larger.

Taking the human mitochondrial genome as an example, several vital proteins are encoded here. Genes include those for cytochrome b, six subunits of the NADH dehydrogenase complex, and three for cytochrome oxidase – all proteins which are instrumental in electron transfer and therefore energy conservation in mitochondria. The genome also contains a gene for a component of ATP synthase, responsible for ATP synthesis. Therefore, these are vital proteins, not just ones peripheral to normal cellular function. However, many of these electron transfer complexes also require the presence of proteins encoded by the nuclear DNA, and therefore the synthesis of a complete and active complex requires the co-ordinated expression of genes from both the mitochondria and the nucleus. Proteins encoded by the nucleus and destined for the interior of the mitochondria will contain special **signalling sequences** which allow the cell to direct the proteins to the right place. It is intriguing that the cell has what appears to be such a complicated mechanism to synthesize these enzyme complexes, but it has been suggested that mitochondria were once prokaryotic in origin and that, therefore, this mechanism is an anomaly created by evolution.

Some degenerative diseases such as Parkinson's disease are thought to be due to defects within the mitochondrial genomes of affected individuals. Such defects are thought to lead to an increase in the oxidative stress within the mitochondria which lowers their production of ATP so vital for cellular function.

Chloroplasts

Again, as seen with mitochondria, chloroplasts of plants contain a circular DNA genome. However, the variation in size between chloroplasts from different species is less pronounced, with most chloroplast genomes falling between 100 and 200 kb. As seen with the mitochondria, many of the genes found here are essential to chloroplast function, with many of the proteins involved in photosynthesis being encoded here, although the complexes once again require the addition of proteins encoded by the nuclear DNA. In addition, many chloroplast genomes also contain large repeated sections, although the significance of this is not known.

Suggested further reading

Barrell, B.G., Bankin, A.T. and Drouin, J. (1979). A different genetic code in human mitochondria. *Nature*, **282**, 189.

Blackburn, E.M. (1991). Telomeres. *Trends in Biochemical Sciences*, **16**, 378–381.

Hammans, S.R. (1994). Mitochondrial DNA and disease. *Essays in Biochemistry*, pp. 99–111. Portland Press.

Jordan, E. and Collins, F.S. (1996). Human genome project: a march of genetic maps. *Nature*, **380**, 111–112.

Stoneking, M. and Soodyall, H. (1996). Human evolution and the mitochondrial genome. *Current Opinion in Genetics and Development*, **6**, 731–736.

Umesono, K. and Ozeki, H. (1987). Chloroplast gene organisation in plants. *Trends in Genetics*, **3**, 281–287.

Wagner, R.P, Maguire, M.R. and Stallings, R.L. (1993). *Chromosomes*. Wiley-Liss.

Zakian, V.A. (1996). Structure, function and replication of *Saccharomyces cerevisiae* telomeres. *Annual Review of Genetics*, **30**, 141–172.

Zakian, V.A. (1996). Telomere functions: lessons from yeast. *Trends in Cell Biology*, **1**, 29–33.

World Wide Web sites of interest

Magpie genome sequencing projects:
http://www.c.mcs.anl.gov/home/genomes/
Human Genome Project information pages:
http://www.ornl.gov/hgmis/home.html
The Dog Genome Project:
http://mendel.berkeley.edu/dog.html

Self-assessment questions

1. What is a bacteriophage?

2. How does one look for the presence of bacteriophages in a sample?

3. Briefly describe the genome of a retrovirus.

4. What is a plasmid?

5. Where in eukaryotic cells, other than the nucleus, is DNA found?

6. What is a nucleosome?

7. What name is given to the ends of chromosomes?

8. Why are mitochondrial genomes so important to cellular function in eukaryotes?

Key Concepts and Facts

- Bacteriophages are viruses that attack bacteria but are important as vectors.

- Bacteriophages have one of three basic structures.

- Bacteriophages have two life cycles: lytic or lysogenic.

- Genome sizes for viruses, bacteria and eukaryotes are very varied between species.

- Retroviruses are RNA-containing viruses.

- Bacteria commonly contain plasmids as well as nucleoid DNA.

- Plasmids are important as gene vectors.

- DNA may move around genomes, for example as transposons.

- Eukaryotic DNA is packaged into chromosomes.

- Extra-nuclear DNA in mitochondria and chloroplasts is very important, as such genomes encode for vital proteins.

Chapter 5
Transcription and RNA

Learning objectives

After studying this chapter you should confidently be able to:

Describe the early stages of the processes of protein synthesis, starting with a gene sequence.

Describe the components of RNA.

Describe mRNA and the modifications made to it.

Describe the structure of tRNA.

Outline the role of rRNA and its synthesis.

Discuss DNA polymerases.

Outline the stages and processes of transcription.

The reason for the existence within organisms of genetic information, or a genome, is to enable a cell to manufacture proteins. Therefore, we shall examine this process further. Not only is such a discussion interesting from an academic standpoint, but if the genes of an organism are going to be manipulated by a molecular geneticist, with perhaps a view to expression of the new gene product in a cell, then it is necessary to understand the processes that take place.

The information encoded by a gene has firstly to be copied into an RNA molecule, which in eukaryotes will take place in the nucleus. This is a process known as **transcription**. Once the RNA has been synthesized, the information can be used to create a protein, a process that takes place on the **ribosomes** of the cell, and is known as **translation**. We will consider the latter process in the next chapter.

Transcription

DNA in many organisms exists as a double-stranded length of nucleotides, and therefore presents us with our first problem. As the two strands have a different order of nucleotide bases, then which is the correct one which contains the genetic information needed? Secondly, as the two strands are held together by interactions between the bases, then the bases are not accessible for complementarity to make a copy, as seen in DNA replication in Chapter 2.

The first problem is solved by having specific areas of sequence which are needed to initiate transcription, such areas of a DNA strand being called **promoters**. Regulation of expression and promoters will be discussed further in Chapter 7. The second problem is solved by the enzymatic machinery that catalyses transcription, as we shall discuss.

RNA: what is it?

RNA (ribonucleic acid), like DNA, is a polymeric nucleic acid, and in fact has the same basic structure as a single strand of DNA, as described in Chapter 2. Like DNA, RNA has a sugar backbone, but instead of deoxyribose the sugar is **ribose**. The second difference is seen when we look at the bases that are used. In DNA the bases are adenine (A), guanine (G), cytosine (C) and thymine (T). In RNA we find the first three of these, that is A, G and C, but thymine is replaced by uracil (U). During RNA synthesis, as will be described below, the order of bases inserted into the growing RNA chain is dictated by the order of bases in the DNA, and uracil will bond to adenine in place of the thymine which was in the DNA second strand. Therefore synthesis of the new RNA will look like the very simplified scheme depicted in Figure 5.1.

Types of RNA

RNA in many cases carries on it the genetic information needed by the cellular machinery to manufacture the appropriate protein and, as we shall see below, the order of the bases on the DNA, and therefore on the RNA, dictates the order of amino acids in that final protein. However, other functions of RNA are also seen, and RNA can be grouped into three types: mRNA, tRNA and rRNA. We will consider these separately below.

mRNA

mRNA, or more fully **messenger RNA**, is the type of RNA that is made and used to decode a gene's information into protein. It is manufactured in the nucleus, but will be exported from the nucleus into the cytosol of the cell, where the information held on it will be used by the protein synthesis machinery to synthesize the new protein.

In general, mRNA species are extremely short-lived, the molecules being very unstable within the cell. As will be discussed in Part Two of this book, this poses problems for the molecular geneticist who might be trying to measure or manipulate mRNA.

DNA

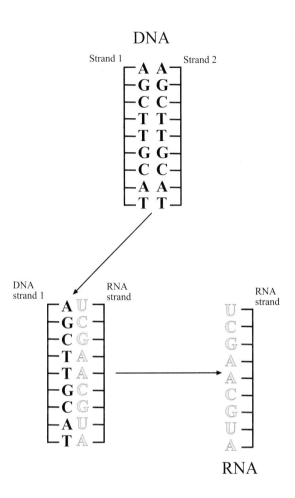

Figure 5.1 *Synthesis of RNA. Strand 1 from the DNA would act as the template here, and the order of the bases in the new RNA is dictated by the order of the bases in the DNA strand. Note thymine (T) is replaced by uracil (U) in the RNA*

RNA

However, as far as the cell is concerned, having mRNA as an unstable molecule is a positive thing. Many genes are expressed only at certain times and in certain amounts, and this expression is very tightly regulated. Therefore, if a cell is not expressing a gene, the mRNA levels will be low. An extracellular signal might then induce the expression of that gene and the mRNA levels will rise. However, the signal might be short-lived and gene expression may need to be stopped. If synthesis of new mRNA is stopped, but the mRNA is stable, then protein synthesis will be able to continue, relatively unchecked. But, if the mRNA is unstable, as soon as mRNA synthesis is reduced, mRNA molecules already in existence will be removed and, as required, protein synthesis will be slowed. However, this is not always appreciated by the researcher who finds their purified mRNA rapidly disappearing in the centrifuge tube!

mRNA, once made, may also undergo many modifications before it is used for protein synthesis. In eukaryotes, genes tend to have introns, or areas of non-coding, as discussed in Chapter 3. These areas have to be removed before translation, or else a whole series

U-RNA is a type of RNA, rich in the base uracil, which is localized in the nucleus of cells. Its function seems to be to aid in the post-transcriptional modification of mRNA. These RNA molecules are alternatively known as snRNA, standing for small nuclear RNA.

of amino acids may be incorporated into the protein which are not required. Areas of consensus sequences around the splice sites, where the intron is to be removed, have been identified, and the mechanism of removal of the intron is known to involve other RNA species called **U-RNA**. Obviously, this is a complex procedure, and one which has to be accurate in ensuring that the complete mRNA message is correct.

As well as the intron being removed, the ends of the mRNA are also modified. At the $3'$ end of eukaryotic mRNA one will usually find a sequence which is rich in adenine bases, a region known as the **poly(A) tail**. Usually the original RNA transcript is modified by a cleavage event, where several bases are removed before the adenine bases are added. This cleavage usually occurs between 10 and 30 bases **downstream**, that is towards the $3'$ end, from a short consensus sequence. This sequence is referred to as a **polyadenylation** signal and commonly would have a sequence that is very similar to $5'$-AAUAAA-$3'$.

Once the RNA has been cleaved, adenine-containing nucleotides are added by an enzyme called poly(A) polymerase, to create a sequence which contains a run of several A units at the $3'$ end of the molecule. This is the poly(A) tail, and if sequencing a gene using a mRNA-derived DNA, the researcher will look for the presence of the poly(A) tail as an indicator of whether the sequence is complete at the $3'$ end. In addition, as mRNA commonly contains this polyadenylation, the presence of a run of A units can be used in the purification of mRNA from all the other species of RNA in the cell. Commonly, a short DNA sequence containing a run of T units is synthesized and then used to capture the mRNA. Under the right conditions the poly(A) tail will hybridize to the poly(T) DNA. If this poly(T) DNA is immobilized, then the RNA species unable to hybridize will be washed away, leaving the mRNA behind. A clever modification to this is to immobilize the poly(T) DNA to magnetic beads. With this system, once the hybridization has taken place and the mRNA has been captured, it can be purified simply with a magnet.

The $3'$ end of the mRNA is not the only one to be modified. At the other end (the $5'$ end) a **cap structure** is added. When the RNA is synthesized, the $5'$ end will be left with a triphosphate, that is three phosphate groups in a line, as seen in Figure 2.4. Firstly a guanine-containing nucleotide is added to this triphosphate, utilizing the $5'$ carbon of the ribose sugar. Once this has been achieved the guanine base is methylated. Therefore the cap structure can be described as being $m^7GpppNpN$-, where m refers to the methylation, 7 to the position of that methyl group on the guanine base, ppp indicates the triphosphate and NpN- the nucleotides at the end of the RNA (see Figure 5.2).

Although the above describes the cap structure of many mRNA molecules, some mRNAs are further methylated on nucleotides at

The terms upstream and downstream are often used to refer to the relative positions of sequences on RNA or DNA molecules. Upstream means towards the $5'$ end, while downstream refers to the $3'$ direction. As sequences are commonly written with the $5'$ end first, on the left, going towards the $3'$ end, upstream can be seen as back to the left of the sequence while downstream means keep reading to the right.

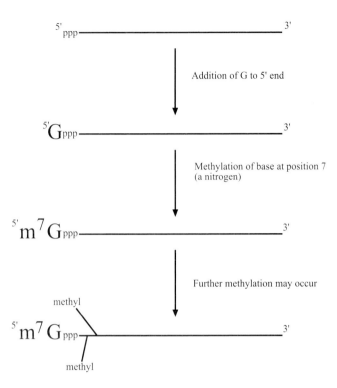

Figure 5.2   *The process of capping the 5′ end of mRNA*

the 5′ end of the chain, although the reason for this remains unclear.

tRNA

tRNAs or **transfer RNA**s are used in the process which actually synthesizes proteins. Their role is simply to capture the right amino acid, bring it to the ribosome and make sure that it is inserted into the growing amino acid chain at the right point. Therefore, one of the major roles of tRNA is to decode the genetic code.

tRNAs are small RNA molecules, typically between 70 and 95 bases long, but they nearly all fold into a similar structure, known as the **cloverleaf**, as depicted in Figure 5.3.

As can be seen from Figure 5.3, the tRNA molecule has several features:

- The **TΨC arm**. This is named after the sequence TΨC, which is usually found along this region of the molecule. Ψ is pseudo-uracil, a pyrimidine-type base.

- The **DHU arm**, or just D arm. This also contains an unusual pyrimidine base, but this time dihydrouracil, hence the name DHU.

- The **optional arm**, otherwise known as the extra or variable arm. The length of this structure can be used to class tRNAs.

Crick first suggested the existence of tRNA in the 1950s, but it was not isolated until 1959 by R. Holley.

Figure 5.3 *The structure of tRNA resembles a cloverleaf*

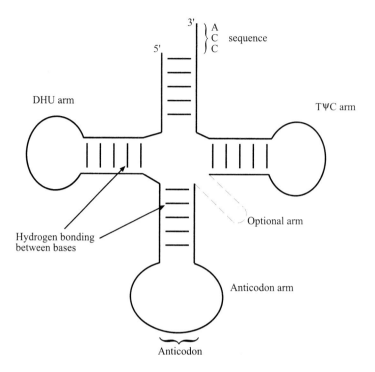

Class I tRNAs have short optional arms of usually five bases or less, while Class II have optional arms which are longer, perhaps 13–21 bases.

However, the crucially important features of the tRNA molecules are the **anticodon arm** and the **acceptor arm**. The latter consists of both ends of the molecule hydrogen bonded together, but the 3′ end contains the sequence 5′-CCA-3′. It is here that the appropriate amino acid is attached for transfer to the ribosome.

The last feature mentioned is the anticodon arm. This contains a sequence of bases which is three nucleotides long, known as the anticodon. This is used to ultimately decode the genetic code, as will be seen later when we consider translation.

tRNAs are transcribed from genes and then, like mRNA, are subject to modification. In eukaryotes, each tRNA is transcribed by a separate gene, although these genes may occur in multiple copies allowing high levels of transcription, and these genes may be clustered together within the genome. In prokaryotes, some genes may contain the sequences of more than one tRNA and the mature tRNAs are released when the precursor transcript is cleaved into sections. This process is catalysed by **ribonucleases** called RNase D and RNase P.

When the sequence of the genes encoding tRNAs are analysed, the 3′ end may not contain the CCA sequence as predicted. These three nucleotides are added by an enzyme called **tRNA nucleotidyl transferase**. Furthermore, the molecules also contain modified bases such as pseudouracil. These are modifications of bases encoded by the gene, with each of the modifications needed being catalysed by a specific enzyme. In fact over 50 different modifications have been reported for tRNAs, including methylations, deamination (removal of an amino group), base rearrangements, and saturation of double bonds. The importance of such changes has been demonstrated, as tRNA molecules which have been synthesized *in vitro* but are unmodified are unable to attach to their relevant amino acid, whereas *in vitro* synthesized modified tRNA molecules are fully functional.

Although the cloverleaf structure is a convenient way of depicting the tRNA molecule, in reality of course it has a three-dimensional structure. Using X-ray diffraction A. Rich and colleagues revealed the three-dimensional structure to resemble an L.

Even though nearly all tRNA molecules are very similar in their overall size and shape there are some exceptions. For example, the mitochondrial tRNAs are somewhat different, but even here similarities are apparent.

> To determine the size of very large complexes, their rate of sedimentation through a dense medium in a centrifuge is commonly used. The value put on this rate of sedimentation is called the sedimentation coefficient or S value, with the unit being the Svedberg unit. Svedberg was a Swede who in the 1920s developed the ultracentrifuge. The S value of a molecule relies on its size as well as its shape.

rRNA

rRNA or **ribosomal RNA** is one of the components of ribosomes, the enzymatic machinery which synthesizes new proteins. Ribosomes are extremely large complexes made up of rRNA and proteins. Prokaryotic ribosomes are typically 2.5×10^6 daltons (Da), with a sedimentation coefficient of 70S, while eukaryotic ribosomes are larger, having a sedimentation coefficient of 80S and a molecular mass of over 4.2×10^6 Da.

Ribosomes can be broken down to two subunit structures, a large and a small subunit. Prokaryotic (70S) ribosomes consist of subunits of 50S and 30S while eukaryotic (80S) ribosomes consist of subunits of 60S and 40S, the compositions of which are listed in Table 5.1.

Table 5.1 *Composition of typical prokaryotic and eukaryotic ribosomes: here mammalian ribosomes are used as a typical example of the eukaryotic system*

Type of subunit	Size	Number of RNA molecules	Sizes of RNA molecules: bases/S	Number of polypeptides
Prokaryotic (large)	50S 1.59×10^6 Da	2	2904 bases/23S 120 bases/5S	34
Prokaryotic (small)	30S 9.3×10^5 Da	1	1541 bases/16S	21
Mammalian (large)	60S 2.82×10^6 Da	3	4718 bases/28S 160 bases/5.8S 120 bases/5S	49
Mammalian (small)	40S 1.4×10^6 Da	1	1874 bases/18S	33

Therefore the functioning of the ribosomes relies on a complex interaction between rRNA and polypeptides, the exact nature of which is still not fully understood. The role of the rRNA is intriguing though. Traditionally it has been thought that catalytic activity within cells is undertaken by the proteins and therefore the rRNA in ribosomes simply must serve as a scaffold on which the proteins attach. However, RNA species have been found elsewhere which appear to partake in their own catalytic activity. The first such example to come to light was an RNA from the ciliate *Tetrahymena* which appeared to self-splice its own introns. Such enzymatic RNA species are called **ribozymes**, and it is thought that the RNA molecules within the ribosomes may also contain such activity.

As can be seen in Table 5.1, each ribosome contains several rRNA molecules, for example the mammalian ribosome has four rRNAs. However, each ribosome has only one copy of each rRNA species. Like all other RNAs, they are encoded by a gene within the genome and their production relies on transcription of those genes. Therefore, it is important that the cell transcribes an equal number of each. To do this, the rRNAs are transcribed from a single transcriptional unit, to create what is called the **primary transcript**. This is a long rRNA precursor, or pre-rRNA. The original gene encodes the rRNAs required and transcription would yield one length of RNA containing all the rRNAs. These would be separated by short spacer sequences. Cleavage would yield immature rRNA species which would then be processed to their final sizes, as depicted schematically in Figure 5.4.

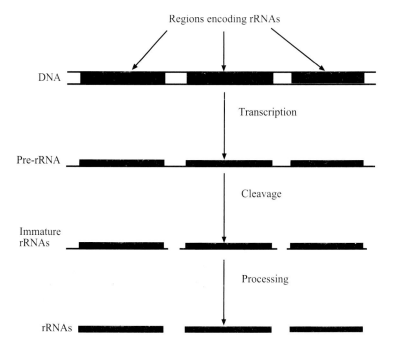

Figure 5.4 *Schematic representation of the transcription and production of rRNA molecules from a single transcriptional unit on the genome's DNA*

The exception to this is one of the mammalian rRNAs, the 5S species, which is encoded separately in the genome.

In rapidly dividing cells the demand for rRNAs is extremely large and, to accommodate this, genomes contain multiple copies of the rRNA transcriptional units. For example, humans have 280 with 2000 copies of the separate 5S rRNA gene.

RNA polymerases

As mentioned above, the first part of the process needed to make an RNA copy of a DNA strand is to open out the DNA double strand, and then to use the order of the DNA bases to guide the formation of the RNA strand, so as the base order created in the DNA strand is totally complementary to the original DNA base order.

These processes are carried out by enzymes known as RNA polymerases. One of the most well studied RNA polymerases is that from *E. coli*. Here, the polymerase is composed of five polypeptide subunits, two α, one β, one β' and one σ. However, this association can exist in two forms: one which is complete, $\alpha_2\beta\beta'\sigma$, known as the **holoenzyme**, and one which is missing the σ subunit, called the **core enzyme**, with the subunit structure $\alpha_2\beta\beta'$. However, it should be noted that more than one type of σ subunit has been identified in *E. coli*, different σ species conferring different specificity to the promoters to which they will bind.

RNA polymerases of eukaryotes, however, are more complex. Here there are three types of polymerase, i.e. I, II and III, which have different roles within the nucleus. Type I is responsible for transcription of ribosomal RNA, while type II transcribes messenger RNA leading to protein synthesis. Type III seems to be responsible for transcription of small RNA species, including tRNAs. As a general rule, these polymerases are larger and more complex than those from prokaryotes, although some of the subunits appear to have similar roles, and even some sequence similarities.

The process of transcription

The process of transcription can be segregated in three phases:

- Initiation
- Elongation
- Termination.

Initiation is a key event in the control of the process, as transcription must not take place randomly on the DNA, but rather gene sequences must be transcribed into RNA. Therefore, initiation of transcription must take place at the correct point, just upstream of the required gene, as discussed further in Chapter 7. Elongation is the process of producing the RNA. Transcription takes place in the

Although transcription takes place in the 3′ to 5′ direction along a gene, when a gene sequence is written down, it is usually the complementary strand in the 5′ to 3′ direction which is shown, which is equivalent to the RNA sequence.

3′ to 5′ direction along the DNA strand, and therefore the new nucleotides are added to the 3′ end of the growing RNA molecule during transcription. Termination, on the other hand, is the end of the process and here, as with initiation, it is important that the transcripts are ended at the correct point along the DNA. Therefore, let us look at each of these processes a little more closely using *E. coli* as a model organism.

Initiation

Initiation must start at the correct point along the DNA and on the correct strand. To enable the cell to achieve this small sequences on the DNA are used which are recognized as start sites. These sequences are known as **promoters**. The promoters are recognized by the polymerase holoenzyme, with its $\alpha_2\beta\beta'\sigma$ subunit structure. It is, in fact, the σ subunit which is responsible for the promoter recognition. How does the polymerase find the correct promoter sequences out of all the DNA? The measured rate constant for polymerase binding is extremely fast, of the order of $10^{10}\,\mathrm{M}^{-1}\,\mathrm{s}^{-1}$, over 100 times faster than that predicted by a random encounter of the polymerase with the DNA. It is likely that the polymerase firstly attaches to the DNA in a rather random way and then moves along it until the correct sequence is found. An analogy to this would be rather like a person in an aeroplane looking for a motorway service station. The pilot may fly around the country for a very long time without going anywhere near a service station. However, it would not be long before they overflew a motorway. Once a motorway has been located, the pilot simply has to fly along it and a service station will appear within a few miles.

The initial protein (polymerase) DNA complex formed is known as a **closed promoter complex**, but it is imperative that the DNA double strand is opened out to reveal the bases before these bases can be used as a template for RNA synthesis. Therefore, one of the first things that the polymerase does is prise apart a region of the DNA double strand, as depicted in Figure 5.5, to create what is referred to as an **open promoter complex**. Elongation can now occur.

Elongation

The rate of reaction of a biological process is often measured. In the example cited in the text, the rate of binding was found to be extremely fast, and gives an indication of the mechanism which might be involved.

Once the open promoter complex has formed, the σ subunit has finished its job and dissociates from the rest of the polymerase complex to leave behind the core enzyme. This core enzyme will now synthesize the new RNA molecule. Most RNA molecules start with pppG or pppA and, unlike for DNA synthesis, a primer is not needed. Once the synthesis is started, the polymerase moves along the DNA double strand, adding ribonucleotides to the 3′ end of the growing RNA and sequentially unwinding the DNA as it proceeds. However, only a small section of the DNA is unwound at any one

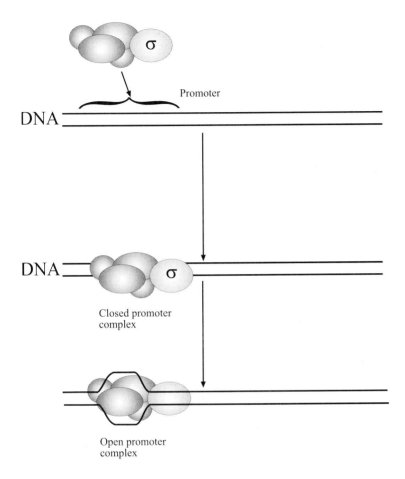

Figure 5.5 *Binding of RNA polymerase to the promoter. The initial complex is a closed promoter complex, but unwinding of the DNA forms an open promoter complex*

Promoter

DNA

DNA

Closed promoter complex

Open promoter complex

moment, and DNA is rewound as it is finished with. Clearly, large molecular restraints prevent large-scale unwinding of the DNA, or nucleotide cleavage would occur, which is undesirable.

Rather intriguingly, the rate of elongation and therefore synthesis of the RNA appears not to be constant. However, both the reason for and the significance of this are not clear.

Termination

In a similar way to initiation, which has to be directed to a particular sequence of DNA, termination must take place at the correct point. It has been found that the DNA sequences around the termination regions of genes are **invariable inverted repeats** i.e. the sequence is symmetrical about a certain point, otherwise known as a **complementary palindrome**. An example would be as shown in Figure 5.6.

This means that the DNA strands are able to hybridize not only to each other, but also to themselves, simply a little further along the chain. Furthermore, the RNA which derives from the DNA

Figure 5.6 *Termination sequences are symmetrical around a point, with the end result being that the RNA formed can form stem-loop structures*

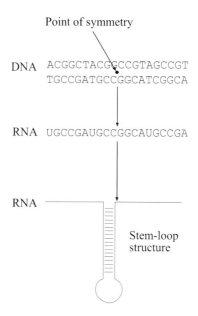

Point of symmetry

DNA   ACGGCTACGGCCGTAGCCGT
      TGCCGATGCCGGCATCGGCA

RNA   UGCCGAUGCCGGCAUGCCGA

RNA

Stem-loop structure

sequence can also self-hybridize, and this will form a structure known as a **stem-loop structure**, as shown in Figure 5.6.

A second feature of termination regions is that the inverted repeat sequences are followed by a run of A units. This is significant when one looks back at the DNA structure (see Chapter 2). As in the DNA strand, A units will be hybridized to U units in the growing RNA strand, but there are only two hydrogen bonds per A/U pair, compared to three hydrogen bonds in a G/C pair. Therefore, if there is a run of A units and therefore A/U pairs, this is a relatively weak attraction.

But how does termination proceed and how do these self-complementary sequences influence termination? It is thought that, as the polymerase reaches the termination point, the stem of

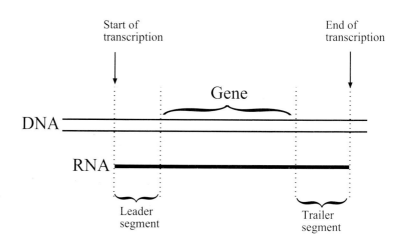

Start of transcription

End of transcription

Gene

DNA

RNA

Leader segment

Trailer segment

Figure 5.7 *The final RNA transcript. As well as the gene of interest, the polymerase transcribes sequences either side, known as the leader segment and trailer segment*

the inverted repeat region is transcribed into RNA, but the formation of a stem-loop structure in the RNA transcript for some reason causes the polymerase to pause or stall. At this point, the RNA is held to the DNA only by the run of weakly bonded A/U pairs. Therefore, the complex is able to fall apart, effectively ending any further transcription.

The form of termination described above is known as **Rho-independent termination**, as a second mechanism has been discovered which involves the activity of a protein called **rho** (ρ). Rho is a large protein of approximately 276 kDa, discovered by Jeffrey Roberts, who was interested in why RNA polymerase transcription of some phages terminated early *in vitro*. Here, in what is called rho-dependent termination, the DNA still contains the inverted repeat sequence but does not contain the run of A units. It is probable that the run of A units and therefore the weak region of attraction between the DNA and RNA are not needed, as the rho protein is responsible for the physical release of the RNA from the DNA. It should be noted here that rho appears to have no association with the polymerase and the two enzymes apparently work independently, unlike the σ initiation factor.

The final transcript

The final transcript produced by the polymerase is usually longer than the gene itself. This is because the promoter, or start site, is upstream of the gene, leaving what is known as a **leader segment** in the RNA before the gene. The length of the leader is very variable, and can be as short as a few nucleotides or as long as several hundreds. Similarly, the termination point is downstream of the end of the gene and therefore it leaves what is called a **trailer segment,** as illustrated in Figure 5.7.

Transcription in eukaryotes

Transcription in eukaryotes is essentially the same process as that described above, starting with an initiation event which ensures that transcription starts at the correct place, followed by an elongation phase, and ending with a termination event, again at the correct region of the DNA. However, the details of these events are different in eukaryotes. To begin with, in eukaryotes there are three types of polymerase, as described above. Each of these will recognize a particular region of the DNA as its unique start site. Polymerase II which transcribes mRNA, for example, uses a consensus sequence of 5'-TATAAAT-3', otherwise known as a TATA box, as will be described further in Chapter 7. Secondly, initiation involves several other proteins known as **transcription factors**. Again using polymerase II as an example, here the transcription factors are called TFIIA, TFIIB, etc. However, a wide variety of transcription factors have been reported, which recognize particular DNA sequences and are themselves perhaps controlled through cell signalling pathways.

Termination of transcription in eukaryotes differs in detail too. Polymerase II can have very long trailer segments, possibly in the region of thousands of bases, whereas polymerase I uses an 18 base-pair sequence approximately 600 bases downstream from the end of the gene. Polymerase III does not appear to use a stem-loop structure to guide termination but does seem to need the presence of a run of A units.

Suggested further reading

Brimacombe, R. and Stiege, W. (1985). Structure and function of ribosomal RNA. *Biochemical Journal*, **229**, 1–17.

Henkin, T.M. (1996). Control of transcription termination in prokaryotes. *Annual Review of Genetics*, 30, 35.

Lee, M.S. and Silver, P.A. (1997). RNA movement between the nucleus and the cytoplasm. *Current Opinion in Genetics and Development*, 7, 212–219.

Rich, A. and Kim. S. (1978). The three dimensional structure of transfer RNA. *Scientific American*, **238**, 52–62.

Ross, J. (1996). Control of messenger RNA stability in higher eukaryotes. *Trends in Genetics*, **12**, 171–175.

Stryer, L. (1995). *Biochemistry*, Freeman. (Chapter 33 in particular.)

Wickens, M. (1990). How the messenger got its tail: addition of poly(A) in the nucleus. *Trends in Biochemical Sciences*, **15**, 277–281.

Self-assessment questions

1. What are the two processes needed to produce a protein from a gene sequence?
2. How does DNA differ from RNA?
3. Why is the instability of mRNA an advantage to the cell?
4. How can a poly(A) tail be advantageous to mRNA purification?
5. How is the structure of tRNA commonly depicted?
6. Where on a tRNA molecule is the amino acid attached?
7. What are the basic differences between prokaryotic and eukaryotic ribosomes?
8. What is the subunit structure of the holoenzyme of RNA polymerase from *E. coli*?
9. In which direction does transcription take place on the DNA?
10. What is the region upstream of a gene at which initiation of transcription takes place?
11. Name two types of transcription termination.

Key Concepts and Facts

- To create a protein from a gene sequence requires the processes of transcription followed by translation.

- RNA contains ribose, not deoxyribose, and the base uracil (U) and not thymine (T).

- Transcription of a gene which encodes a protein yields messenger RNA (mRNA).

- mRNA is modified once produced: (1) by the addition of a poly(A) tail; (2) by the addition of a cap structure; and (3) by removal of any introns.

- tRNA brings the amino acids to the ribosomes.

- The structure of tRNA is referred to as a cloverleaf.

- Ribosomes carry out the process of translation, and are composed of rRNA and proteins.

- Prokaryotic ribosomes are 70S while eukaryotic ribosomes are 80S.

- RNA is produced by RNA polymerases.

- Transcription has three phases: initiation, elongation and termination.

- Initiation starts at the promoter region of the gene.

- Termination may be rho-dependent or rho-independent.

Chapter 6
Translation and the genetic code

Learning objectives

After studying this chapter you should confidently be able to:

Explain how the information in a gene sequence leads to the correct amino acid sequence in a protein.

Outline the work which led to the elucidation of the genetic code.

List the features of the genetic code which allow it to work.

Describe how tRNA shows specificity to its particular amino acid.

Outline the process of translation.

In Chapter 5 the process of transcription was discussed, where the DNA encoding a particular product was unzipped and an RNA copy of one of the DNA strands was synthesized. It may be that the RNA copy is the final product required by the cell, such as an RNA molecule which will be incorporated into a ribosome, i.e. rRNA. However, a great many RNA molecules are further used to direct the synthesis of a protein. This RNA is the messenger RNA (mRNA). Therefore we see that the cell uses the scheme shown in Figure 6.1 to synthesize its proteins.

Here, we will discuss the second part of this process, that is the process of translation – the synthesis of the polypeptide molecule. However, we know that a protein or polypeptide is simply a string of amino acids which has been added together. Thus a protein may be depicted as in Figure 6.2. Therefore we have to have mechanisms

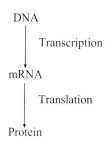

Figure 6.1 *Flow of genetic information from DNA*

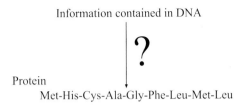

Information contained in DNA

?

Protein

Met-His-Cys-Ala-Gly-Phe-Leu-Met-Leu

Figure 6.2 *A protein is a sequence of amino acids, determined by the DNA that encodes it*

in the cell whereby the information held by the DNA is used to order the amino acids within the protein. But what is it about the DNA which enables it to be used as a source of information? As discussed in Chapter 2, DNA comprises a string of nucleotides, each with the presence of a particular base. So here we have an order of bases in the DNA, and an order of amino acids in the protein. Therefore, the bases in some way code for the amino acids in the protein. But how is this achieved?

Decoding the DNA

Instrumental work in this area has been achieved by many researchers, but notably **Francis Crick**, **Sydney Brenner** and **H. Gobind Khorana**. The problem, in simplified terms, is that the DNA has a choice of four bases which could be inserted in any one position (defined by the nucleotide). However, a protein could have a choice of any one of 20 amino acids which could be inserted in any one position along its length. Therefore, a single base could not determine the location of a single amino acid. Perhaps two bases would do? However, there are only 4×4 or 16 combinations of two bases, and therefore again this would not work. However, if each amino acid was determined by a run of three bases then the combinations of bases possible would be $4 \times 4 \times 4$ or 64. But how could this be verified experimentally?

Two experimental procedures were required to test the hypothesis that the coding of RNA was based on three bases. Firstly, RNA needed to be synthesized with a known sequence. And, once the base sequence could be dictated by the researcher, the question remained as to what the resulting protein sequence would be. Secondly, translation needs to be possible in a cell-free extract so that synthesized RNA sequences could be tested. The first problem was solved with the isolation of polynucleotide **phosphorylase** in 1955 by Severo Ochoa and Marianne Grunberg-Manago. This enzyme catalyses the reaction:

$$(RNA)_n + \text{ribonucleoside diphosphate} \rightarrow (RNA)_{n+1} + P_i$$

where n denotes the number of bases in the RNA. Of interest here is the fact that this enzyme requires no DNA template. Therefore by manipulation of the nucleotides added, the researcher could manipulate the resultant sequence of the RNA produced.

The second procedure, that of translation in the absence of the cell in what is referred to as a **cell-free system**, was devised by

Severo Ochoa received the Nobel prize for his work in 1959. In 1985 he became Professor of Biology in Madrid, which is where he had received his MD in 1929.

> **Marshall Nirenberg** received the Nobel prize for his work in 1968, 2 years after the completion of the genetic code.

Marshall Nirenberg and Heinrich Mattaei in 1961 using *E. coli* as a source of translational machinery.

Therefore, artificial RNA could be made and tested in the laboratory. For example, RNA was synthesized with only U, giving poly(U) with the sequence:

5′-U-U-U-U-U-U-U-U-U-U-U———3′

and then tested to see which amino acid was incorporated. In this case it would be phenylalanine. Similarly poly(A) led to the incorporation of only lysine and poly(C) led to the incorporation of only proline. Therefore, if the bases are coding in threes as suggested, the code words for phenylalanine, lysine and proline would be UUU, AAA, and CCC, respectively.

However, the results above still do not tell us the length of the code words. If the RNA is -UUUUUUU- all we know is that a run of Us results in the incorporation of phenylalanine, not the length of that run of Us. It could still be UU, or UUU, or UUUU, etc. Therefore, to further probe the coding, RNA molecules were produced with alternate bases, such as -UGUGUGUGUGUGUGUGUGUGU-. If the code words are two bases in length, the codes are either UG or GU, but either way it results in the incorporation of only one repeating amino acid. However, if the code words are three bases long, the codes are either UGU or GUG and these are alternate. Therefore, the resulting protein should have alternating amino acids. When this experiment was performed the result was the protein sequence Cys-Val-Cys-Val-Cys-Val-Cys-Val-.

This can be explained if the RNA and protein are aligned as in Figure 6.3.

Therefore, Cys must be encoded for by UGU while GUG encodes Val. Similarly, poly(AG) with the sequence AGAGAGAGAGAG resulted in the protein Arg-Glu-Arg-Glu-, where Arg must be encoded by AGA and Glu by GAG.

Experiments further took advantage of RNA sequences in which three bases were repeated, as seen in Figure 6.4. Here, the sequence AAG is repeated, giving the three base repeats of either AAG, AGA or GAA. If the bases were truly read off three at a time the resulting proteins would only have one amino acid incorporated, but three such proteins would result, depending on the first base used to decode the message. The three potential starts and the results are shown in Figure 6.4.

Other combinations used were poly(UUC) giving either phenylalanine, serine or leucine incorporated, and poly(UUG) giving leucine, cysteine or valine incorporated.

At a similar time, other researchers such as Nirenberg in 1964

UGU	GUG	UGU	GUG	UGU	GUG	U
Cys	Val	Cys	Val	Cys	Val	

Figure 6.3 *An alternate base sequence leads to an alternate incorporation of amino acids if the coding requires three bases*

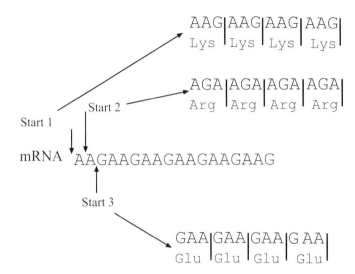

Figure 6.4 *RNA sequences with three bases repeating result in polypeptides of only one amino acid, but three different such polypeptides will be produced*

used binding studies to probe the genetic code. Here it was found that certain trinucleotides promoted the binding of tRNA species to ribosomes and, using these results together with those from the cell-free experiments described above, the genetic code was elucidated.

There are several points that need to be highlighted here:

- **Colinearity**. The genetic code has colinearity. This means that the order of the bases in the DNA corresponds directly to the order of the amino acids in the protein.
- The codewords. The genetic code does indeed require a sequence of three bases to determine the incorporation of a single amino acid into the growing protein. The three base codeword is known as a **codon**. Clearly there are 64 possible codons and only 20 amino acids to code for. Therefore, several codons may code for the same amino acid. An extreme example here is serine which is coded for by six codons: UCU, UCC, UCA, UCG, AGU and AGC. Codons which code for the same amino acid are known as synonyms and the genetic code is said to be degenerate. Generally most synonyms only vary in the last base used. The codons xxC and xxU always code for the same amino acid. The full genetic code is given in Table 6.1.
- Start? Clearly, if the genetic code is going to be read like we read a sentence of a book, we need to know where to start and stop. In English we use capital letters and full stops. What does the genetic code use? As a start signal all proteins start with the amino acid methionine. In prokaryotes the first amino acid is a modified methionine, that is **formyl-methionine** (fMet), while in eukaryotes it is simply methionine. However, methionine is found in proteins in other places, not just at the beginning. Therefore the translational machinery has to find the correct methionine to start and not just any in the sequence. In

Table 6.1 *The genetic code: in this table, the first position of the codon is read down the far-left column, the second codon position along the top row, and the third position down the far-right row*

	U	C	A	G	
U	UUU Phe	UCU Ser	UAU Tyr	UGU Cys	U
	UUC Phe	UCC Ser	UAC Tyr	UGC Cys	C
	UUA Leu	UCA Ser	UAA … STOP	UGA … STOP	A
	UUG Leu	UCG Ser	UAG … STOP	UGG Trp	G
C	CUU Leu	CCU Pro	CAU His	CGU Arg	U
	CUC Leu	CCC Pro	CAC His	CGC Arg	C
	CUA Leu	CCA Pro	CAA Gln	CGA Arg	A
	CUG Leu	CCG Pro	CAG Gln	CGG Arg	G
A	AUU Ile	ACU Thr	AAU Asn	AGU Ser	U
	AUC Ile	ACC Thr	AAC Asn	AGC Ser	C
	AUA Ile	ACA Thr	AAA Lys	AGA Arg	A
	AUG *Met*	ACG Thr	AAG Lys	AGG Arg	G
G	GUU Val	GCU Ala	GAU Asp	GGU Gly	U
	GUC Val	GCC Ala	GAC Asp	GGC Gly	C
	GUA Val	GCA Ala	GAA Glu	GGA Gly	A
	GUG Val	GCG Ala	GAG Glu	GGG Gly	G

prokaryotes, the start methionine codon, that is AUG, is preceded by a purine-rich region which base-pairs with a sequence within the rRNA of the ribosomes (the **Shine–Dalgarno sequence**: see below). In eukaryotes the AUG codon is probably but not always the first AUG found in the sequence. This suggests that the sequence surrounding the initiation AUG codon is also important in some cases.

Often when a gene has been cloned and sequenced, as discussed in Part Two, research will need to identify the start of the encoding region, and often mistakes have been made where the wrong methionine has been identified as the start, although the location of a Shine–Dalgarno sequence will help here.

- Stop? The end of the translated region is determined by one of three codons which basically encode 'stop'. These are UAA, UAG and UGA. Of course, if mutations take place in the DNA which create one of the stop codons instead of an amino acid encoding codon, the results may be catastrophic as the resultant protein will be shorter than intended. Such proteins would be referred to as being **truncated**, and are very likely to be non-functional. As with the start of the encoding section, researchers often need to find the end of the encoding region when cloning. This is easier as it will be the first stop codon encountered while reading along the sequence from the start codon. The region between the start methionine and the first stop codon is referred to as the **open reading frame** (ORF).

Although AUG is usually the first codon used to incorporate methionine and indicate the start of translation, GUG is sometimes used in prokaryotes. It should be noted that GUG also codes for valine.

- Universal? The genetic code is virtually universal. Genes taken from plants can be decoded by animal cells, while genes from prokaryotes can be decoded by eukaryotic systems. Without such a universal nature to the code, genetic manipulation and genetic engineering would be much more difficult than it is. However, the genetic code is not totally universal. Some codons in mitochondrial systems differ from the nuclear sequences. For example, as described above, UGA usually codes for a stop codon, but in mitochondrial translation it codes for the incorporation of tryptophan. It has been reported too that ciliated protozoa have slight alternations from the universal code, but generally such differences are rare and are the exception rather than the rule.

Translation

Loading of the tRNA

The role of transfer RNA (tRNA) is to transfer a particular amino acid to the site of protein synthesis, and ensure that the correct amino acid is incorporated into the growing protein at the correct point. Therefore, the first step is to bond the correct amino acid to the correct tRNA. This in fact is a two step process, as shown in Figure 6.5.

Firstly the amino acid has to be activated. The amino acid and ATP are used to form an intermediate known as **aminoacyl-AMP** or alternatively aminoacyl adenylate. This intermediate then reacts with the appropriate tRNA to create what is referred to as a **charged tRNA**, that is the tRNA with its own specific amino acid attached to the CCA terminus of the RNA.

The reaction between the amino acid and the tRNA is catalysed by a group of enzymes called **aminoacyl-tRNA synthetases**. There is, in fact, at least one synthetase for each amino acid, and it is here

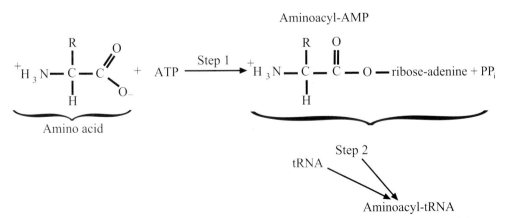

Figure 6.5 *The reactions catalysed by aminoacyl-tRNA synthetase. R denotes the side chain of the amino acid*

Figure 6.6 *Schematic representation of the double sieve hypothesis*

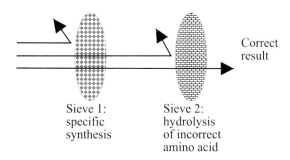

Sieve 1: specific synthesis

Sieve 2: hydrolysis of incorrect amino acid

Correct result

Table 6.2 *Amino acids used by the two classes of aminoacyl synthetases*

Class	Amino acids used
Class I	Arg, Cys, Gln, Glu, Ile, Leu, Met, Trp, Tyr, Val
Class II	Ala, Asn, Asp, Gly, His, Lys, Phe, Ser, Pro, Thr

that the specificity of the reaction occurs. Remember, it is vitally important that the correct amino acid is associated with the correct tRNA. But how is this achieved?

The explanation of how this works has been dubbed the **double sieve hypothesis**. It is thought that the synthetase firstly has a specificity towards both the correct tRNA and the correct amino acid, and so only the correct match is catalysed. This would be the first sieve. However, several amino acids are very closely related structurally. For example, alanine and glycine only differ by the presence or absence of a single methyl group (CH_3 instead of H). Therefore, mistakes are bound to happen, and mistakes can not be made here, because it is the tRNA which helps to direct the amino acid incorporation into the protein. If the tRNA is charged incorrectly, the wrong amino acid will be incorporated. However, it has been found that the synthetases also contain a hydrolytic activity, and if the wrong amino acid has been added to the tRNA then it will be cleaved from the tRNA. This is the second sieve. A schematic representation of this is shown in Figure 6.6.

Aminoacyl-tRNA synthetases are grouped into two classes depending on the presence of a particular sequence of amino acids within them. In general terms, class I synthetases are used to charge tRNAs with the larger and more hydrophobic amino acids, while the smaller amino acids use class II synthetases. The amino acids used by the two classes are shown in Table 6.2. Interestingly, there are ten in each class.

Codons and anticodons

Once the tRNA has been charged with the correct amino acid the second part of the tRNA which we need to discuss is the region known

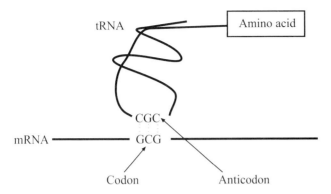

Figure 6.7   *Identification of a codon by the anticodon of appropriate tRNA*

Table 6.3   *Possible unusual bonding at the third or wobble position of the codon–anticodon*

Base found in anticodon (position 1)	Possible bases that can pair in the codon (position 3)
C	G
G	U or C
U	A or G
A	U
I	U, C or A

as the **anticodon**. In the discussion above we saw that the RNA can be read in groups of three bases known as codons, and it is the order of the three bases which determines the amino acid incorporated. The anticodon of the tRNA is also three bases, but these are complementary to those on the RNA, as depicted in Figure 6.7.

However, the complementarity between the codon and the anticodon is not always perfect. It was proposed by Crick in 1966 as the **wobble hypothesis** that more than one codon could be recognized by a tRNA anticodon. This is because bonding can take place between bases which do not usually come together. This unusual bonding takes place at the third position of the codon, the so-called **wobble position**. Many anticodons also use an unusual base called **inosine**. Bonding at the other two positions of the codon is as expected, but the unusual bonding patterns possible at the third positions are summarized in Table 6.3.

Therefore, by allowing wobble, the cell needs few different tRNAs to decode all 64 codons. In fact some cells can use as few as 31 different tRNA species.

The process of translation

The process of translation itself takes place on the ribosomes. Normally ribosomes exist as dissociated subunits in the cytoplasm

Inosine is a deaminated form of guanine, where an NH_2 group has been removed from the carbon at the second position around the ring.

of the cell. Therefore the first step in the process is to assemble the ribosomes into a catalytic unit. As with transcription, the process can be separated into three parts:

- Initiation
- Elongation
- Termination.

The process has been well characterized in *E. coli* and therefore, firstly, the steps here will be considered separately using this as a model organism.

Initiation

The process of translation must begin at the correct place along the mRNA and, as discussed above, protein synthesis always starts with the incorporation of a formyl-methionine (or methionine in eukaryotes). How does this occur? The 30S subunit of the ribosome will bind to the mRNA at a site just upstream of the first methionine codon (or initiation codon). This ribosome binding site has been identified and found to have the consensus sequence:

$$5'\text{-AGGAGGU-}3'$$

This sequence is known as the Shine–Dalgarno sequence and probably works by base-pairing with the 16S rRNA in the ribosomal subunit. The 30S subunit will now move along the mRNA and locate the initiation codon where an initiation complex can form. Here the appropriate charged tRNA, i.e. tRNA bound to formyl-methionine, joins the complex with the anticodon base-pairing with the codon (see Figure 6.8). The synthesis of the protein has now started as the first amino acid is in place. However, in theory, protein synthesis could continue to proceed in either direction, upstream from the first methionine or downstream. In practice, protein synthesis always takes place from the methionine towards the carboxyl terminus of the protein. That is, protein synthesis is always in the $N \rightarrow C$ direction, with the methionine (or formyl-methionine) being at the N-terminal end. In prokaryotes, as the methionine is formylated, the process is only possible in this direction anyway.

Initiation also involves other proteins known as **initiation factors**. Three have been identified in *E. coli*, known as IF1, IF2 and IF3. IF2 binds also to GTP which is hydrolysed later in the process, driving the dissociation of IF1 and IF2 from the complex.

Elongation

The initiation complex is now joined by the large 50S ribosomal subunit. This is associated with the hydrolysis of GTP bound to IF2. The result is a complete ribosome with mRNA attached, and with

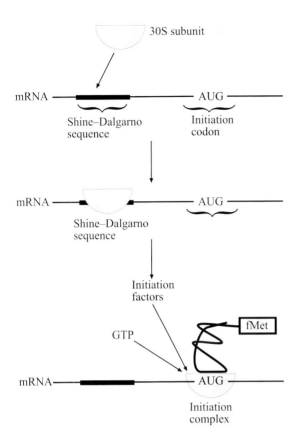

Figure 6.8 *Formation of the initiation complex at the beginning of translation. The 30S subunit binds to the Shine–Dalgarno sequence and moves along the mRNA to the AUG initiation codon. tRNA then associates with the mRNA*

the fMet-tRNA base-paired to the AUG initiation codon. However, in the completed ribosome there are, in fact, two tRNA binding sites. These are known as the **peptidyl-site** or **P-site** and the **aminoacyl-site** or **A-site**. At the beginning the P-site is occupied by the fMet-tRNA, as depicted in Figure 6.9, while the A-site lies in line with the second codon which needs decoding.

As with initiation, other proteins are also involved in the elongation of the protein. These are **elongation factors** known as EF-Tu and EF-Ts. EF-Tu is a G protein and has the capacity to bind GTP. This GTP is hydrolysed to GDP in a cycle. A simplified version of the G protein cycle is shown in Figure 6.10. EF-Tu in the GTP-bound state helps to position the next charged tRNA into the A-site of the ribosome. Once this has occurred the GTP is broken

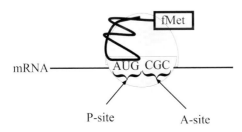

Figure 6.9 *The initiation complex of translation. An fMet-tRNA aligns with the P-site while the A-site is empty, awaiting the arrival of the next charged tRNA*

Figure 6.10 *Simplified scheme showing the G protein cycle*

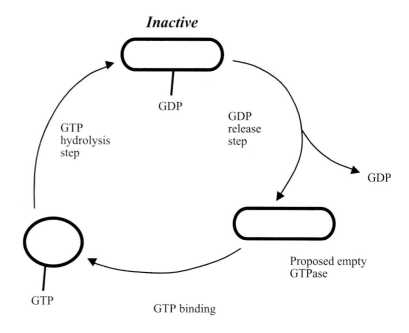

Inactive

GDP

GTP
hydrolysis
step

GDP
release
step

GDP

GTP

Proposed empty
GTPase

GTP binding

G proteins, or guanine nucleotide binding proteins, are commonly found as control proteins in many cell signalling cascades. They have the capacity to bind GTP and hydrolyse this to GDP. They are commonly activated and deactivated depending on whether GTP or GDP is bound (see Figure 6.10). Common examples are the trimeric family which controls enzymes such as adenylate cyclase and phospholipase C, and the monomeric family which includes the oncogene product RAS.

down to GDP and EF-Tu dissociates to start the next round of elongation. The second elongation factor, EF-Ts, is responsible for the dissociation of GDP from EF-Tu, to allow another GTP to bind and to allow the cycle to continue.

Therefore, after EF-Tu has introduced a second charged tRNA into the ribosome, this time in the A-site, there are now two amino acids in close proximity, and in an order dictated by the base sequence of the mRNA. A peptide bond is now formed between the two amino acids, catalysed by an enzyme activity within the ribosome called **peptidyl transferase**. Secondly, the tRNA which brought the fMet to the P-site in the first place has finished its job and we now need to remove it. This is catalysed by a second enzyme activity in the ribosomes called **tRNA deacylase**. This breaks the bonds between the amino acid and the tRNA, freeing the tRNA so it may be recharged and recycled.

We now have the first tRNA detached from its amino acid in the P-site and a tRNA attached to a short peptide chain, that is the two amino acids joined together, in the A-site. This is depicted in Figure 6.11. The first tRNA is released and we therefore need to slide along the mRNA to the next codon, a process known as **translocation**. The result of this is that the tRNA attached to the peptide chain now enters the P-site and we have a free A-site, ready for the entry of the next charged tRNA. This situation is totally analogous to the earlier situation where the first tRNA charged with the formyl-methionine had entered the P-site. Therefore we see that the process is a cycle which can be repeated, but with each round of the process the ribosome with its growing peptide chain moves down the mRNA by one codon, a distance of three bases.

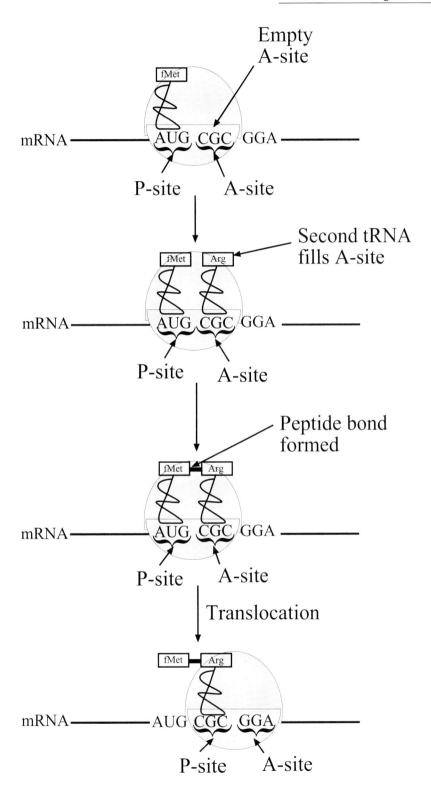

Figure 6.11   *The elongation cycle of translation*

Translocation is controlled by another elongation factor, called EF-G. This too is classed as a G protein, cycling between a GTP-bound form and a GDP-bound form. The GTP-bound form drives the translocation step while hydrolysis of the GTP drives the release of the EF-G.

Termination

As discussed above, there are three codons which signal the end of translation: UAA, UAG and UGA. Therefore, when one of these aligns with the A-site of the ribosome, translation must finish (see Figure 6.12). This time, instead of a charged tRNA entering the A-site, there are proteins known as **release factors** which enter. One release factor, RF1, recognizes the stop codons UAA and UAG while a second, RF2, recognizes UAA and UGA. The releasing factors activate the peptidyl transferase activity of the ribosome, resulting in the release of the new polypeptide which has been synthesized. Termination also appears to involve the 16S RNA of the ribosome itself as well as a third release factor, RF3.

Translation in eukaryotes

The process of translation in prokaryotes as described above is very similar to that in eukaryotes. However, there are a few differences worth noting.

- Ribosomes: These are 80S ribosomes composed of 60S and 40S subunits.
- Initiation: In eukaryotes there is not a Shine–Dalgarno sequence, but the mRNA does have a cap structure which is used for ribosome binding. Usually, but not always, it is the first AUG (methionine) codon which is used as the initiation codon.
- Initiation factors: Many more are involved in eukaryotic translation, denoted by eIF. The formation of the initiation codon also requires the hydrolysis of ATP.
- First amino acid: The first amino acid is an unmodified methionine, not formyl-methionine.
- Monocistronic: The mRNA in eukaryotes only has one start site as it codes for only one protein. In prokaryotes, the mRNA may have several start sites and code for several proteins.
- Termination: Requires the hydrolysis of GTP and only a single release factor, eRF.

It should be borne in mind that many proteins when purified do not actually start with a methionine at the N-terminal end. Often a cleavage of the protein has taken place and the first few amino acids are removed, perhaps because they were originally involved in a signalling process.

Polysomes

In both prokaryotes and eukaryotes it has been found that the same mRNA molecule may be translated by several ribosomes at the same time. A piece of mRNA associated with several ribosomes is

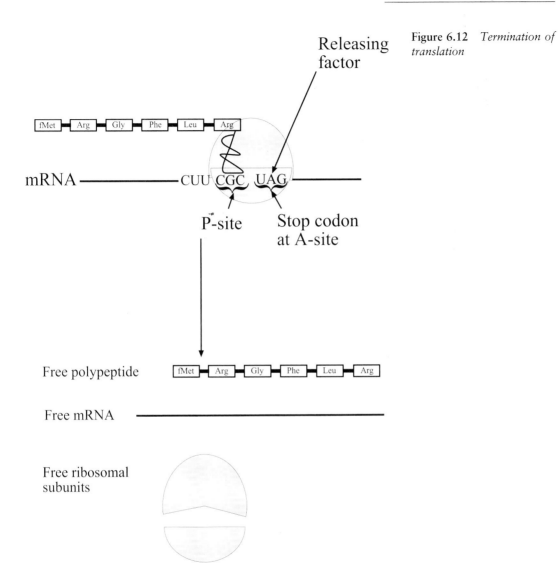

Figure 6.12 *Termination of translation*

known as a **polysome**. The ribosomes nearest to the initiation codon have the shortest polypeptide chains, while the ribosomes nearest the termination site have been translating a longer stretch of mRNA and therefore have longer polypeptide chains attached. This is shown in Figure 6.13.

Suggested further reading

Carter, C.W. Jr. (1993). Cognition, mechanism and evolutionary relationships in aminoacyl-tRNA synthetases. *Annual Reviews of Biochemistry*, **62**, 715–748.

Figure 6.13 *Structure of a polysome – several ribosomes all translating a single mRNA*

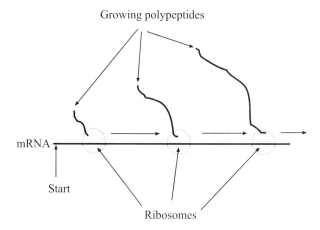

Growing polypeptides

mRNA

Start

Ribosomes

Green, R. and Noller, H.F. (1997). Ribosomes and translation. *Annual Reviews of Biochemistry*, **66**, 679–716.

Merrick, W.C. (1992). Mechanism and regulation of eukaryotic protein synthesis. *Microbiology Reviews*, **56**, 291–315.

Moras, D. (1992). Structural and functional relationships between aminoacyl-tRNA synthetases. *Trends in Biochemical Sciences*, **17**, 159–164.

Noller, H.F. (1991). Ribosomal RNA and translation. *Annual Reviews of Biochemistry*, **60**, 191–227.

Proud, C.G. (1992). Protein phosphorylation in translational control. *Current Topics in Cell Regulation*, **32**, 243–369.

Sachs, A.B., Sarnow, P. and Hentze, M.W. (1997). Starting at the beginning, middle and end: translation initiation in eukaryotes. *Cell*, **89**, 831–838.

Stryer, L. (1995). *Biochemistry*. Freeman. (Chapter 34 in particular.)

Self-assessment questions

1. Which two procedures were required to test the hypothesis that the genetic code was read as a sequence of three bases?
2. What amino acid sequence would be synthesized from the gene sequence UGUGUGUGUGUGUGUGU and why?
3. What does colinearity refer to when discussing the genetic code?
4. What is a codon?
5. What amino acid invariably starts a newly synthesized protein in:
   (a) eukaryotes;
   (b) prokaryotes?
6. What are the three stop codons?
7. Which hypothesis explains the specificity of the binding of tRNAs to amino acids?

8. In which direction does the synthesis of proteins take place?
9. What are the factors involved in the termination of translation called?
10. What is a polysome?
11. How is the structure of inosine related to that of other bases found in nucleic acids?

Key Concepts and Facts

- Translation uses mRNA as a source of information to make a new protein.

- Translation takes place on ribosomes.

- A gene sequence is read off in words three bases long, called codons.

- RNA molecules synthesized with defined sequences were instrumental in unravelling the genetic code.

- The genetic code shows colinearity.

- The gene sequence has defined start and stop codons.

- The first amino acid incorporated into a protein is methionine or formyl-methionine.

- The charging of a tRNA with its amino acid has to be accurate – a process carried out by aminoacyl-tRNA synthetases.

- The anticodon of the tRNA decodes the sequence by binding to its appropriate codon.

- Translation has three phases: initiation, elongation and termination.

- Protein synthesis takes place in the N to C direction.

Chapter 7
Control of gene expression

Learning objectives

After studying this chapter you should confidently be able to:

Explain how to find the site of protein binding on a DNA strand.

Explain aspects of the control of prokaryotic gene expression.

Describe the structure of operons.

Outline the negative and positive control of operons.

Explain aspects of the control of eukaryotic gene expression.

Describe common structures of transcription factors.

As we saw in Chapter 5, it is vital that transcription starts at the correct part of the DNA molecule to ensure that the gene is copied correctly to the RNA transcript and that the correct sequence is used to make either the protein via translation or the RNA molecule with its own function. However, is it not only important to ensure that the correct part of the DNA is transcribed, but also vital that the genes are transcribed only when required. The majority of genes, but not all, are transcribed and translated only occasionally, and may be described as being **inducible**. A few genes appear to be transcribed continuously, and as such their expression is described as **constitutive**, and these genes are dubbed **house-keeping genes**, an example being the gene for α-actin. Such house-keeping genes are often used by molecular geneticists as an internal control, especially when studying inducible genes.

DNase protection experiments

Once it has been established that a protein such as a **polymerase** attaches to the DNA molecule and catalyses transcription, how does the researcher identify the particular part of the DNA sequence which is recognized by that protein? One of the methods is known as a **DNase protection experiment**. DNase, or to give it its full name deoxyribonuclease, is an enzyme which

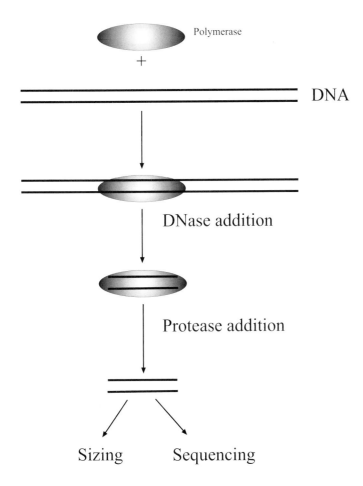

Figure 7.1   *DNase protection experiment. Sequential addition of DNase and protease will reveal the region of DNA protected by the polymerase or other DNA binding protein*

catalyses the removal of nucleotides from DNA. Therefore the experiment will proceed along the following lines.

1. DNA fragment and DNA binding protein (here we will say a polymerase) are incubated together.
2. The mixture is DNase treated. Here, all the exposed DNA will be broken down into component nucleotides. Parts of the DNA which have bound to the polymerase will be protected and not destroyed by the DNase.
3. DNase is washed off.
4. A protease is added to remove the protein component (polymerase).
5. The remaining DNA can be sized by electrophoresis and sequenced to find the exact region on the original DNA which bound to the polymerase.

This scheme is illustrated in Figure 7.1.

Figure 7.2 *Positions of promoter sequences in* E. coli

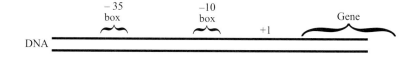

François Jacob and Jacques Monod shared the Nobel prize for their work in 1965.

Prokaryotic gene expression

Promoter regions of prokaryotes

In prokaryotes the polymerase holoenzyme binds to a region upstream of the gene known as the **promoter**. In *E. coli* two regions of DNA are found to be important: one 10 bases upstream (position −10) of the gene and another 35 bases upstream. This is illustrated in Figure 7.2. The −10 box is often called the **Pribnow box**, after David Pribnow who first described the comparisons of several *E. coli* and phage promoters. Both these regions have defined consensus sequences. The −10 box has a consensus sequence of -TATAAT-, while the −35 box has the sequence -TTGACA-. Of course, not all promoters have these exact sequences, an example being that of the lactose operon, which has the two sequences -TATGTT- (−10) and -TTTACA- (−35), but all will be very similar. Interestingly, not all variations are allowed, however, and some alterations of the consensus sequence will completely destroy polymerase binding.

Operons

Operons and their control was first proposed by François Jacob and Jacques Monod. It was realized that the control of several related genes was co-ordinated, and that the products of these genes appeared together. This led to the proposal that these genes were linked and their expression was controlled from a single point on the DNA. Such a set of contiguous genes with co-ordinated control is termed an operon. The first described and most well-defined operon was the **lactose operon**. Here, three genes which are needed by the bacterium to switch from the metabolism of glucose to the metabolism of lactose are in one operon. These genes are:

- *LacZ*: Encodes for β-galactosidase, used for the conversion of lactose to galactose and glucose, which are further used in the metabolism of the cell. Also converts lactose to allolactose.

- *LacY*: Encodes for galactoside permease, used to transport the lactose into the cell.

- *LacA*: Encodes for galactoside transacetylase, with an unknown function.

The three genes are contiguous on the DNA, and are therefore transcribed into a single **polycistronic** message, using a single promoter as a control point. This is illustrated in Figure 7.3.

As can be seen in Figure 7.3, there is another gene, namely *lacI*. This codes for a protein called the **lac repressor**. This protein is a

Polycistronic refers to the fact that the message created is a transcript from more than one gene. Cistronic here is simply a synonym for gene. Eukaryotic messages are invariably monocistronic, that is, from only one gene.

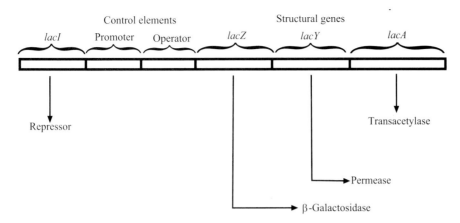

Figure 7.3   *The lactose operon*

tetramer of 37 kDa subunits, with each subunit having a binding site for an inducer. Structural studies of the repressor polypeptide show that each subunit has an axis of two-fold symmetry. A wild-type cell may only contain a few molecules of the repressor and, therefore, when it was originally isolated, the researchers used cells which were over-expressing the repressor gene.

   The last part of the lac operon is the control region, comprising a promoter to which the polymerase attaches and an operator to which the repressor may attach.

   Having described the structure of the lactose operon, we shall now describe its control. In the absence of lactose and in the presence of another source of metabolic fuel such as glucose, there will be an absence of the lactose inducer in the cell. The repressor protein will be synthesized by expression of the *lacI* gene, and this protein will bind to the operator region of the lac operon. Such binding prevents the functioning of the polymerase and therefore transcription is prevented. This scheme is illustrated in Figure 7.4a. The repressor appears not to prevent the binding of the polymerase to the DNA, but prevents the formation of an open promoter complex, so stopping transcription from proceeding.

   However, in the presence of lactose, the cells will contain a lactose inducer. This inducer will bind to the binding sites on the repressor subunits, and in so doing will alter the conformation of the repressor protein. The repressor is then unable to bind to the operator region of the operon and prevent transcription (Figure 7.4b). Therefore, in the presence of lactose, the genes are able to be expressed, producing the proteins that are necessary for the metabolism of lactose.

   What is the inducer that causes this effect? In the laboratory the traditional inducer has been IPTG (isopropyl-thiogalactoside). However, in *E. coli* the physiological inducer is **allolactose**. This is formed by a transglycosylation of lactose. This reaction is rather oddly catalysed by β-galactosidase, which is one of the genes

(a)

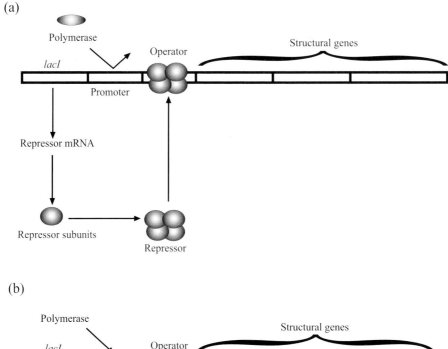

(b)

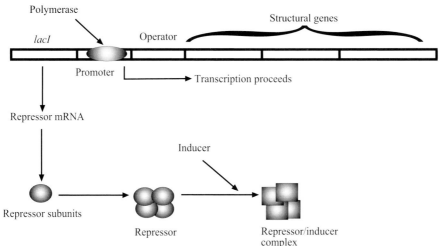

Figure 7.4   *Regulation of the lac operon. (a) In the absence of lactose, the repressor binds to the operator region and prevents transcription. (b) In the presence of lactose, allolactose is formed which binds the repressor. This complex is unable to bind to the operator and so transcription is able to proceed*

encoded by the operon itself. Therefore the question arises as to where the β-galactosidase comes from in the first place to enable the inducer to be formed which then induces synthesis of the β-galactosidase enzyme itself. The answer comes when it is realized that *E. coli* will never be devoid of the enzyme β-galactosidase, and that the low level of the enzyme found in the cells is enough to form some allolactose. Once the operon starts to be expressed, the new β-galactosidase will allow a faster rate of allolactose formation.

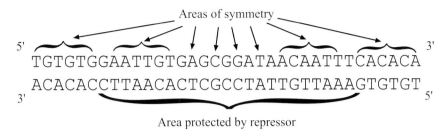

Figure 7.5 *Nucleotide sequence of the lactose operator. Note the areas of symmetry*

In a similar way to that already seen with polymerase binding to DNA, the binding of the repressor to the operator has been found to have an extremely fast rate constant (of the order of $10^{10}\,\mathrm{M}^{-1}\,\mathrm{s}^{-1}$). Once again, it is likely that the repressor binds loosely and randomly to the DNA, and then moves along it in search of the correct operator region.

The repressor subunits have been found to contain an axis of symmetry, and this is not surprising when the sequence of the operator region is studied. This too has a symmetry, as shown in Figure 7.5.

The control of the lactose operon as described above can be referred to as a form of negative control. That is, in the absence of lactose the operon is suppressed. However, the operon is also under positive control too. Here, the cells are effectively sensing and acting on the absence of glucose to induce the operon, enabling the cells to switch to a new metabolic fuel. Cells will usually preferentially use glucose as a source of fuel and therefore, in the presence of both glucose and lactose, there is no need to switch on expression of the lactose operon, and cells will simply continue to use glucose. This is referred to as **catabolite repression**. However, it is when glucose runs low that cells need to express operons such as the lactose operon. Therefore cells need to sense the lack of glucose as a control signal.

This control is based around the levels of cAMP in cells, cAMP being a well-known and well-characterized second messenger molecule in cells. cAMP in both prokaryotes and higher organisms is often dubbed a **hunger signal**, and in the slime mould *Dictyostelium*, cAMP is used as an extracellular signal controlling slime formation.

The presence of glucose on the outside of the *E. coli* cell causes the intracellular concentrations of cAMP to be low, but how do cAMP levels control the lac operon? cAMP binds to a protein called CAP, or **catabolite gene activator protein**. CAP is a dimer of 22 kDa subunits, with each subunit able to bind to both DNA and cAMP. In the absence of cAMP, CAP is unable to bind to DNA and thus cannot influence the level of lac operon expression. Therefore, amid high levels of glucose, cAMP is low and CAP has no effect. However, when the concentration of glucose falls, the level of cAMP in the cells increases and cAMP binds to CAP to form a

cAMP is cyclic adenosine monophosphate (or, more correctly, adenosine 3′,5′-cyclic monophosphate).

Second messengers in cells are molecules which are produced in cells in response to extracellular signals, such as hormones. Molecules on the outside of the cell are referred to as first messengers, while their 'message' is relayed inside the cell by second messengers. cAMP is a classic example, produced by the enzyme adenylate cyclase (otherwise known as adenylyl cyclase).

Figure 7.6 *Binding of the cAMP-CAP complex to the lactose operon. This facilitates the binding of the polymerase*

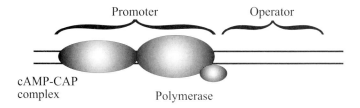

cAMP-CAP complex. CAP undergoes a conformational change and is then able to bind to DNA. The cAMP-CAP complex actually binds to the promoter site of the operon adjacent to the binding site of the polymerase (Figure 7.6). It aids in the binding of the polymerase to the promoter as well as stimulating transcription itself.

The arabinose operon

The lactose operon is not the only such system found in prokaryotes. Other well-characterized operons include the arabinose operon. Here once again the cells are preparing themselves to use an alternative source of fuel, this time arabinose. This can be converted to xylulose 5-phosphate by three enzymes: arabinose isomerase, ribulokinase and ribulose 5-phosphate epimerase. These enzymes are coded for by three contiguous genes called *araA*, *araB* and *araD*, respectively. These are arranged in an operon as shown in Figure 7.7.

The control of the arabinose operon is in many ways very similar to that of the lactose operon, except for various details which are worth a mention. Firstly, there are two operator regions, $araO_1$ and $araO_2$. Secondly, the product of the *araC* gene is not a repressor like that of the *lacI* gene, but rather a **control protein** (C protein).

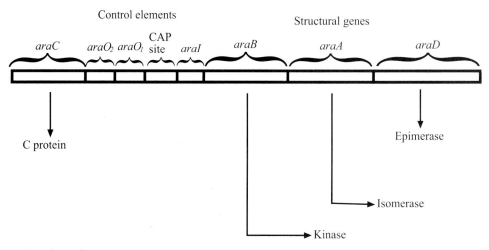

Figure 7.7 *The arabinose operon*

The expression of C protein is from the opposite direction from the *BAD* genes, and is controlled by the operator O_1. Under low levels of C protein, its transcription and translation proceeds, but as levels of C protein rise it binds to *araO₁* and stops its own transcription. Therefore, the levels of C protein are **auto-regulated**. In the absence of arabinose other C protein molecules bridge across the *araO₂* and *araI* control regions, forming a loop in the DNA and preventing the transcription of the *BAD* genes. Hence, here C protein is acting as a repressor, in the same way as the lactose repressor.

However, if arabinose is abundant, arabinose binds to the C protein, altering its conformation. It is now able to bind to *araO₁* and *araI*. No DNA loop is formed and transcription is able to proceed. Here C protein is acting as a positive control. Therefore, with the arabinose operon, the same protein (C protein) acts as both a negative and a positive control.

The second influence on the control of the arabinose operon is once again the cAMP-CAP complex. As with the lactose system, the cAMP-CAP complex signals the lack of glucose availability and binds to the promoter region, aiding the functioning of the polymerase to enhance transcription of the genes.

Operons for synthetic pathways

The operons described above both encode for series of enzymes involved in the breakdown of metabolic fuels, but other operons encode for enzymes involved in synthetic pathways. Examples here include operons for tryptophan, histidine and phenylalanine synthesis. The tryptophan operon is shown in Figure 7.8.

In this operon there are sites which act as promoters and an operator and, in addition, the tryptophan operon is under the control of a repressor protein, but this time the repressor is coded for by a gene remote from the rest of the operon. This is the *trpR* gene. Binding of tryptophan to the repressor enables it to bind to the operator and prevent transcription. Therefore, when tryptophan

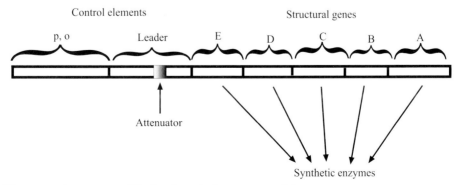

Figure 7.8   *The tryptophan operon. The key here is the presence of the attenuator*

is plentiful, the production of enzymes capable of making more is prevented.

The second mechanism of control here is the use of an **attenuator** or controlled termination site. In prokaryotes there is no spatial separation of transcription and translation. Therefore, translation can begin before transcription has been completed, and this fact helps in the control of the tryptophan operon. The transcript produced starts with a leader sequence of 162 nucleotides, before the E gene starts. Part of the leader is translated. The leader sequence also contains the attenuator region. This region contains two areas of sequence with a two-fold axis of symmetry, one which is rich in G/C bases and one which is rich in A/T bases.

Thus the transcript of the leader sequence is able to adopt a secondary structure, and it is translated before the transcription of the mRNA is completed. Close examination of the amino acid sequence encoded by the leader sequence reveals that at positions 10 and 11 there are two tryptophans, as shown in Figure 7.9. Therefore successful completion of translation of this sequence relies on the presence of tryptophan, and remember that the enzymes being produced here are responsible for tryptophan production. Hence, in the presence of tryptophan, the ribosome successfully translates the leader sequence, and the mRNA can take up a particular secondary structure which interferes with transcription and transcription will stop. In the absence of tryptophan, when the ribosome reaches the part of the leader mRNA where tryptophan is required to continue translation, the ribosome will stall as tryptophan will not be available for it to continue. The mRNA can then adopt a different secondary structure which does not interfere with transcription. Under these conditions, transcription will be completed, the synthetic enzymes will be produced and the levels of tryptophan replenished.

Similar leader sequences are identifiable in other operons too. In the histidine operon leader there is a consecutive run of seven histidines. In the phenylalanine operon there is a run where seven out of nine consecutive amino acids are phenylalanine, and clearly the same mechanisms are shared by these operons.

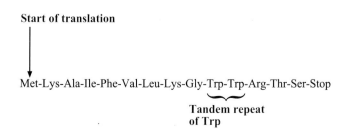

Figure 7.9 *Leader sequence of the tryptophan operon, highlighting the repeated tryptophans*

Eukaryotic gene expression

Eukaryotic gene expression is different from that of prokaryotes in many respects. Firstly, transcription and translation are both temporally and spatially separated due to the presence of the nuclear membrane, and therefore control such as that described above for the tryptophan operon is impossible. Secondly, eukaryotic mRNA is always **monocistronic**, each gene having its own transcription control.

Promoter regions of eukaryotes

The promoters for many genes in eukaryotes have been characterized. Polymerase II recognizes a sequence approximately 25 nucleotides upstream from the transcription start site. This is known as the TATA box and has the sequence 5′-TATAAAT-3′. Many promoter regions also have additional areas of influence further upstream. One such area is the CAAT box with a consensus sequence of 5′-GGNCAATCT-3′, while another is the GC box with the consensus sequence 5′-GGGCGG-3′. Both these boxes are found between nucleotides −110 and −40, as shown in Figure 7.10.

Polymerase I appears to use a site which straddles the transcription start site, running from nucleotides −45 to +20. Promoters for polymerase III are even more unusual, and in fact lie within the transcribed gene. These 50-nucleotide-long regions are called **internal control regions**.

Enhancers

Sequences elsewhere on the DNA can also have a great influence on the activity of the promoters. These sequences are called enhancers. Enhancers can be several thousand bases away from the gene itself. They may be upstream or downstream of the gene, can be on either DNA strand and in either orientation. Some enhancers may be found in the introns of the genes themselves. The positions in which enhancers can be found are depicted in Figure 7.11.

Many enhancers, however, are found to be tissue-specific. They may exert a large influence in one tissue but in another tissue the expression of a gene may not be influenced at all by the enhancer. The enhancer may only work in tissues in which particular specific proteins are expressed.

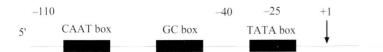

Figure 7.10 *Features that may be found in eukaryote promoters*

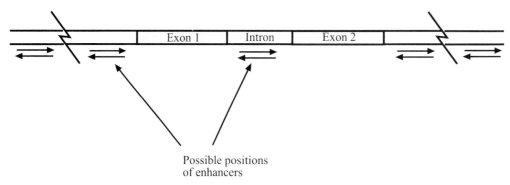

Figure 7.11 *Possible positions and orientations of enhancers: they may be upstream, downstream or even within the gene*

Transcription factors

Expression of genes in eukaryotes relies on the participation of a group of proteins known as transcription factors. These were discussed briefly in Chapter 5. When polymerase II initiates transcription it requires the involvement of several other proteins. Initiation actually starts with a transcription factor called TFIID binding to the TATA box of the promoter. It is able to do this efficiently because part of the TFIID is a 30 kDa component known as the TATA-box binding protein (TBP). TFIIA binds next, followed by TFIIB. TFIIE and polymerase II bind finally, to create a basal transcription apparatus. Although transcription can now occur, other transcription factors may bind to this complex and exert an influence.

Clearly, then, in eukaryotes transcription is greatly influenced by many proteins which come under the label of transcription factors. Many of these proteins share structural similarities. For example, DNA binding proteins may contain one of the following motifs:

- Helix-turn-helix: These polypeptides are so called because within their structure they have two α-helices separated by a sharp turn. This turn is brought about by the presence of four amino acids which preferentially take up this conformation. DNA binding proteins in eukaryotes and prokaryotes may contain such structures. For example, the Trp repressor protein contains a helix-turn-helix motif.

- Leucine zipper: As the name suggests, such proteins contain domains rich in leucines. In fact, leucines reside at every seventh position along a stretch of about 35 amino acids. The polypeptides fold into α-helices with the leucines down one face of the helix. These proteins then dimerize to enable DNA binding. Examples of such proteins include GCN4 found in yeast, which activates the transcription of over 40 genes encoding enzymes used in biosynthetic pathways and **CREB** (cAMP response element binding protein) which is under the control of cAMP levels in cells.

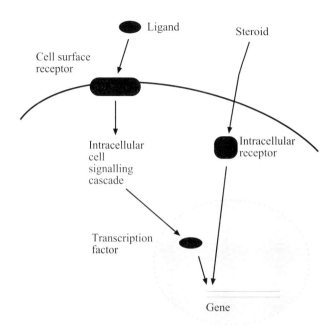

- Zinc fingers: These polypeptides have a structural motif which comprises a 30 amino acid domain which folds into both a β-sheet and an α-helix to resemble a finger, but with a zinc binding region incorporated within it. These proteins contain the consensus sequence:

$$-X_3-Cys-X_{2-4}-Cys-X_{12}-His-X_{3-4}-His-X_4-$$

where X is any amino acid and the subscript numbers denote the number of such amino acids. It is the Cys and His residues which bind to the zinc atom. Examples of such proteins include the Zif268 transcription factor found in mice which has three zinc fingers, and the SP1 protein which is known to bind to the GC box.

Lastly, transcription factors may be under the control of a cell signalling cascade, possibly starting at the cell surface. For example, as discussed above, the CREB transcription factor is controlled by the levels of cAMP in cells. The level of cAMP will be controlled in turn by the activity of the enzyme which synthesizes it, that is adenylate cyclase (adenylyl cyclase), as well as by enzymes which break it down, such as phosphodiesterase. The activity of enzymes such as adenylate cyclase is controlled by hormones and their perception by their particular receptors. Other signalling from receptors through the interior of the cell to the nucleus may involve **phosphorylation cascades** such as the **MAP kinase pathway**. An example here is when relatively high levels of insulin are added to cells. Series of kinases are sequentially activated by their phosphorylation by other kinases, finally result-

MAP kinases (mitogen activated protein kinases) were originally reported to be kinases activated in response to the addition of mitogen to cells. However, recent research has shown that such kinases and kinase cascades in which MAP kinases are found are involved in many responses, particularly stress responses, of a variety of cells, ranging from those of plants to higher mammals.

ing in the activation of a transcription factor and the elevation of transcriptional activity.

Alternatively, hormone receptors may be found inside the cell. Steroids are able to permeate the cell membrane and are perceived by receptors which may reside in the cytoplasm of the cell or even in the nucleus. These receptors may be associated with heat shock proteins, but essentially the binding of the hormone to the receptor ultimately results in the alteration of transcriptional activity. A very simplistic scheme of such cell signalling pathways is given in Figure 7.12.

Suggested further reading

Greenblatt, J. (1991). RNA polymerase-associated transcriptional factors. *Trends in Biochemical Sciences*, **16**, 408–411.

Hancock, J.T. (1997). *Cell Signalling*. Longman (AWL). (For further details on cell signalling cascades and the components involved, including cAMP.)

Jacob, F. and Monod, J. (1961). Genetic regulatory mechanisms in the synthesis of proteins. *Journal of Molecular Biology*, **3**, 318–356.

Kim, J.L., Nikolov, D.B. and Burley, S.K. (1993). Co-crystal structure of TBP recognising the minor groove of a TATA element. *Nature*, **365**, 520–527.

Latchman, D.S. (1995). *Eukaryotic Transcription Factors*, 2nd edn. Academic Press.

Self-assessment questions

1. How does one identify areas on a DNA strand where a protein may bind?
2. What is an operon?
3. Why is the RNA transcript from the lactose operon described as polycistronic?
4. What is the natural inducer of the lactose operon and which enzyme catalyses its formation?
5. What is the second messenger which controls CAP of the lactose operon?
6. How does the function of C protein of the arabinose operon differ from that of the repressor of the lactose operon?
7. Which cellular structure in eukaryotes ensures that transcription and translation are spatially and temporally separated?
8. What is an enhancer?
9. List three common protein structures found in eukaryotic transcription factors.
10. What reaction is carried out by the enzyme adenylate cyclase?

Key Concepts and Facts

Background Facts
- Many genes are under tight regulation of expression.

- DNase protection experiments enable the protein/DNA binding sites to be determined.

- DNA regions which bind to proteins and the proteins involved usually show some symmetry.

Prokaryotes
- Promoters in prokaryotes often contain two areas of consensus sequence.

- Bacterial genes may be contiguous in operons.

- The lactose operon is under both positive and negative control.

- C protein of the arabinose operon auto-regulates its own expression.

- Some operons are under the control of an attenuator region.

Eukaryotes
- The promoter regions of eukaryotes also have identifiable consensus sequences.

- Enhancer regions may also influence the rate of gene expression.

- Transcription is controlled by transcription factors.

- Structures have been defined for many transcription factors.

- Many transcription factors are controlled by cell signalling cascades.

Chapter 8
Inheritance

Learning objectives

After studying this chapter you should confidently be able to:

Outline the experiments of Gregor Mendel.

Explain the patterns of inheritance which result in Mendel's simple ratios.

Draw Punnett squares to determine inheritance ratios.

Explain why Mendel's rules are not followed in the inheritance patterns of many genes.

Gregor Mendel and his breeding experiments

As discussed in Chapter 1, the acknowledged father of modern genetics probably is Gregor Mendel, a monk who carried out simple but elegant breeding experiments. His results were published in 1866, but mostly ignored until the turn of the century until similar experiments were carried out by Hugo De Vries in the Netherlands, Carl Correns in Germany and Erich von Tschermak in Austria.

Mendel had decided to study the characteristics of the pea plant, and this proved to be a good choice, better than his later choice of Hawkweed, which yielded inconsistent results that did not support his earlier conclusions. In his experiments Mendel chose seven features of the pea plant which were easily seen and, fortunately for him, were inherited in a simple manner. These features were:

1. The height of the plants.
2. The flower colour.
3. The flower position, being either axial or terminal.
4. The seed colour.
5. The seed coat texture, either smooth or wrinkled.
6. The shapes of the pea pods, either smooth or indented.
7. The pod colour.

In his experiments Mendel removed the stamens of the flowers to stop self-fertilization and then used a brush to transfer the pollen

Table 8.1 *Typical results obtained by Mendel in his first breeding experiments*

Characteristic being studied	Numbers of each type obtained	Ratio
Height	787 tall/277 short	2.84 : 1
Seeds	5474 round/1850 wrinkled	2.96 : 1
	6022 yellow/2001 green	3.01 : 1
Pods	882 inflated/299 constricted	2.95 : 1
	428 green/152 yellow	2.82 : 1
Flowers	705 purple/224 white	3.15 : 1
	651 axial/207 terminal	3.14 : 1

from one plant to another's stigma, and then harvested the seeds. He first made sure that the plants he was breeding from were pure-breeding and then he crossed two pure-breeding individuals together to get the F_1 generation. Two F_1 plants were then crossed to get the F_2 generation and the characteristics of these recorded. Results typical of those he obtained are shown in Table 8.1.

As can be seen from the results in Table 8.1, most of the ratios of the characteristics that Mendel was studying were approximately 3 : 1. The brilliance of Mendel's work was the interpretation that he put on these ratios. He realized that a simple explanation could account for such a recurring ratio and he drew up the scheme depicted in Figure 8.1.

In this experiment the chosen feature is the height of the plant, which is represented by the letter 'T'. Mendel explained that the pure-breeding tall plant would contain two genetic particles which

> The genotype of an organism refers to the genetic make-up of that particular individual. For example, it might carry two genes for tallness and therefore would have the genotype *TT*. The phenotype refers to the way the individual looks, that is with respect to the particular feature of interest, for example whether the individual is tall or short.

Mendelian inheritance

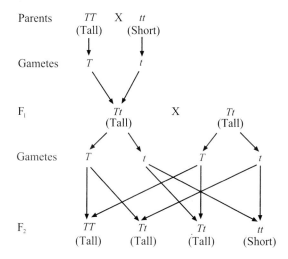

Figure 8.1 *Inheritance pattern of a simple Mendelian trait, showing the genotypes and phenotypes of the individuals and the resulting 3 : 1 ratio*

Homozygous means that the individual contains two alleles which are the same, for example TT or tt would be homozygous for tallness or lack of tallness, respectively. Heterozygous means that the individual has one of each allele, for example Tt.

led to tallness. The individual genetic markers which led to the **phenotypic** characteristic are referred to as **alleles**. We could denoted the tallness allele by the large 'T', and therefore genetically the plant could be represented as *TT*. This would be a **homozygous** individual (see sidebox), that is containing two alleles that are the same. The small pure-breeding plant would therefore contain two genetic particles for smallness, denoted by lower case letter 't's and therefore would be *tt* genetically. The breeding of these together would be the donation of one genetic particle from each plant to create the new genetic plant. The tall plant had no option but to donate a T particle and the small plant had no option but to donate the t genetic particle. Therefore the new plant, the F_1 generation, would be genetically *Tt*, that is, it is **heterozygous**. Mendel discovered that all these plants which contained both a genetic particle for tallness and a genetic particle for smallness were in fact tall. He cleverly suggested that one of the genetic particles may have a dominance over the other and therefore the plant preferentially expressed the feature which was coded for by the **dominant** particle. Of course, Mendel was suggesting this hypothesis long before the discovery of DNA and gene structures. The genetic particle which was not seen in the phenotype was said to be **recessive**. Note that when a dominant and a recessive come together the dominant is always written first; hence the heterozygous form would be written as Tt.

The further breeding of these F_1 generation plants together created the F_2 generation, in which there were three tall plants to every one short plant. As can be seen from Figure 8.1, one F_2 plant would be genetically *TT* and therefore phenotypically tall, while another two plants would have the genotype *Tt*, and also be phenotypically tall, therefore giving a total of three tall plants. The only other possible combination of the genetic particles is *tt*, giving one small plant. Therefore, Mendel's $3:1$ ratio can be explained.

It was fortunate for Mendel that each of the characteristics that he had chosen to study were under the control of a single gene, or genetic particle. This **monogenic** inheritance can be used to explain the inheritance of many characteristics in organisms. Mendel extended his studies to look at the inheritance of two such characteristics at the same time, that is **digenic** inheritance. Such an inheritance pattern can be seen in Figure 8.2.

However, Figure 8.2 highlights the difficulty in drawing out such an inheritance pattern in this manner, and therefore commonly such genetic inheritance is represented in the form of a **Punnett square**. This representation was first used by a British geneticist called R.C. Punnett.

Here, the gametes from the male plant are entered in the top row, while the gametes from the female are entered in the left-hand column. The rest of the rows and columns are filled out by simply repeating those gametes along and down, respectively, but as above,

Mendelian inheritance of two genes

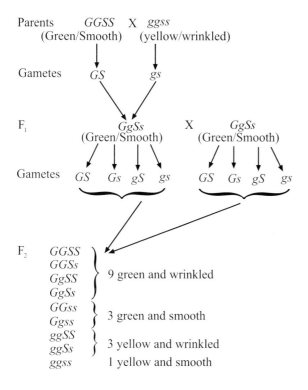

Figure 8.2 *Inheritance pattern for two simple (digenic) traits, showing the resulting 9 : 3 : 3 : 1 ratio*

Table 8.2 *A Punnett square using the data from Figure 8.2*

Female/male	GS	Gs	gS	gs
GS	GGSS	GGSs	GgSS	GgSs
Gs	GGSs	GGss	GgSs	Ggss
gS	GgSS	GgSs	ggSS	ggSs
gs	GgSs	Ggss	ggSs	ggss

the capital letter always precedes the small letter; hence *GgsS* would never be written, rather it would be denoted by *GgSs*. The phenotypes are therefore relatively easy to see and the numbers of each can quite easily be totted up. Any genotype which is *GG* or *Gg* will give the green phenotype, *SS* or *Ss* the smooth phenotype, while yellow or wrinkled will only appear if the genotype is *gg* or *ss*, respectively. Here, the Punnett square confirms the 9 : 3 : 3 : 1 ratio seen in Figure 8.2. This 9 : 3 : 3 : 1 ratio can also be mathematically derived assuming that the alleles are inherited independently. Each separate allele will give rise to a 3 : 1 ratio and 3 : 1 × 3 : 1 as a matrix gives us a ratio of 9 : 3 : 3 : 1. Such 3 : 1 and 9 : 3 : 3 : 1 ratios are looked for when studying unknown alleles to determine if simple Mendelian inheritance is taking place.

Such simple breeding experiments led Mendel to postulate his two laws or principles:

Mendel's first law. Often referred to as the **principle of segregation**, this law refers to the fact that two members of a pair of genes, or alleles, will separate from each other on meiosis and that one half of the gametes formed will carry one gene or allele while the other half of the gametes will carry the other gene or allele.

Mendel's second law. This law, commonly referred to as the **principle of independent assortment**, expands upon the first law by saying that during the formation of gametes, the separation of a pair of genes or alleles will be independent of a second pair of genes. Clearly, if the two genes studied are carried on the same chromosome, then independent separation is not a guaranteed event.

We now know, of course, that the genetic particles Mendel was referring to are, in fact, genes.

Exceptions to the rules

Although many genes follow very well the inheritance patterns laid down by Mendel, many genes don't and if they don't there are several reasons why inheritance is deviating from these simple rules. Some of the these reasons are detailed below.

Incomplete dominance

Incomplete dominance will be seen when Mendelian inheritance patterns appear to be followed but neither allele being studied has dominance over the other. When the two alleles end up in the same individual, the phenotype seen is a mixture of the two original phenotypes. The classic example of this was seen with the work of Carl Correns. He was studying the flower colour of, for example, the carnation, and found that on breeding homozygous red flowering plants (RR) with homozygous white flowering plants (rr) all the F_1 generation, expected to be heterozygous (Rr) and therefore red, were in fact pink. Further breeding of the F_1 generation to get the F_2 generation yielded ratios approaching $1:2:1$ of red : pink : white flowers (see Figure 8.3). Here, the explanation is that the red flowers are homozygous (RR), the white flowers are also homozygous (rr) but the pink flowers are heterozygous (Rr) and, furthermore, show both phenotypes of the parents as a mixture.

Co-dominance

Co-dominance is in many ways similar to incomplete dominance but, instead of a mixture of phenotypes presenting, here both

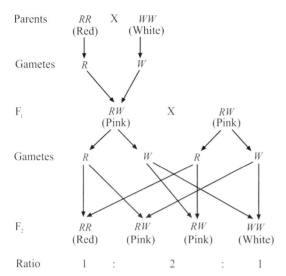

phenotypes are seen together. An excellent example of co-dominance is seen with the human blood grouping. The MN blood group refers to the presence of a glycoprotein on the red blood cell surface and there are two forms, encoded for by two alleles L^M and L^N. Many individuals only show the M form and the underlying genetics would show them to be $L^M L^M$. Conversely, many individuals only show the N form and would be $L^N L^N$ genetically. However, if an individual is genetically $L^M L^N$, then both glycoproteins would be seen and their blood group would be MN. Neither allele dominates and, therefore, the alleles are referred to as being co-dominant.

Multiple alleles

Human blood grouping again serves as a good illustration of this exception to Mendelian thought. The ABO blood grouping is determined by the presence of three different alleles, I^O, I^A and I^B but an individual only carries two. An A individual would carry at least one I^A allele, but no I^B allele, and therefore genetically could be $I^O I^A$ or $I^A I^A$, and a blood group B individual would be $I^O I^B$ or $I^B I^B$. The AB blood group would arise from only $I^A I^B$ while O grouping has to be $I^O I^O$ genetically. Therefore, more than two alleles can contribute to the genetics of the ABO blood grouping, and this is referred to as multiple allelism.

Another good example of this phenomenon is the colouring of the peppered moth, *Biston betularia*. Here, the colouring is determined by the presence of two alleles, but again in a population three alleles encoding colour have been seen, m, M and M'. These alleles also show a dominance hierarchy, as M' is dominant to m, but M is dominant over M'.

Traditionally, the peppered moth, *Biston betularia*, was seen with a light mottled colour. However, today in urban areas, most peppered moths are dark melanic forms. These darker moths are more easily camouflaged against the modern urban background and therefore tend to survive. The darkening of the moths over the decades is an example of what has been termed 'industrial melanism'.

Figure 8.4 *Inheritance pattern of the Manx cat, showing the 2 : 1 ratio and the lethal combination that results in stillbirth*

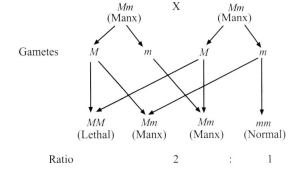

Homozygous individuals for the Manx characteristic of lack of a tail are impossible to obtain, as the MM combination of alleles is lethal and such cats would be stillborn. Therefore to breed Manx cats, heterozygous Mm cats need to be crossed.

Lethal combinations

In some Mendel-type experiments the breeding of two heterozygous individuals would lead to a ratio of 2:1. This is because one combination of alleles would be a fatal combination. A classic example of this is seen with the Manx cat. An individual cannot be homozygous for the Manx characteristic, as individuals that carry this genetic form are stillborn. Therefore, the breeding chart would look like Figure 8.4. As can be seen, there are two ways of obtaining *Mm*, the Manx phenotype, and only one way of obtaining the normal phenotype, *mm*, and hence the ratio of 2:1.

Sex-linked genes

Most of the genes of an organism are carried on chromosomes which can be passed to any individual in the next generation and such chromosomes have no influence on the sex of the individual. These chromosomes are referred to as autosomes. If the gene is carried on an autosome, the inheritance pattern is referred to as being **autosomal**. However, certain chromosomes determine the sex of some organisms and these are referred to as the **sex chromosomes**. In humans, there are two sex chromosomes, denoted as X and Y. As in typical Mendelian inheritance, we all carry two copies of the sex chromosomes, but it is the type of those we carry which determines our sex. In humans, all males carry one X and one Y chromosome, and are therefore XY. Females carry two Xs and are therefore XX. Such inheritance has a profound effect on inheritance patterns. For example, anything carried by the Y chromosomes can never be found in the female, and such an inheritance pattern is referred to as being Y-linked. Alternatively, if a gene is carried by the X chromosome, only one copy of it can ever be carried by a male. Therefore, an X-linked recessive characteristic will be seen in a male as it will have no complementary gene to counter it. Therefore, X-linked characteristics are often seen in males and rarely in females, unless they are dominant characteristics of course. A typical X-linked inheritance pedigree is shown in Figure 8.5.

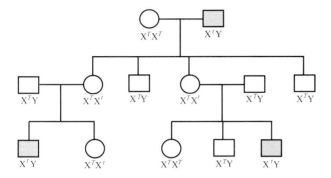

Figure 8.5 *A simple pedigree for a recessive X-linked gene for three generations. Squares denote males, circles females, and shaded shapes afflicted individuals*

Such inheritance patterns are relatively easy to spot in pedigree charts, as they are more common in males than females and they often skip a generation. Common traits which are inherited in such a way include some forms of colour blindness and haemophilia (as seen with the British Royal Family), along with more rare diseases such as some forms of chronic granulomatous disease (CGD).

Abnormalities with respect to the presence or absence of the sex chromosomes themselves can lead to disease states. In humans four main variants are reasonably common:

- XO: only one X chromosome is present. This is known as **Turner's syndrome** where the individuals are sterile females, and usually short in stature.

- XXY: an extra X chromosome as well as a normal male XY. This is known as **Klinefelter's syndrome**, and sufferers are sterile males but may show some female characteristics.

- XXX: an extra X chromosome as well as a normal female XX complement. These people are known as **metafemale** and are also sterile.

- XYY: an extra Y chromosome as well as the normal male XY. These individuals appear not to be sterile, and at one time it was thought that they were prone to violent tendencies.

Other examples of sex determination in an individual by its complement of sex chromosomes include many insects where the female is XX but the male is XO, that is having only one X chromosome and nothing else. In birds, many reptiles and moths the females are heterozygous, ZW, while it is the males that are homozygous, ZZ.

Sex-limited and sex-influenced patterns

Some genetic patterns of inheritance are not directly due to the presence of the gene on one of the sex chromosomes but are affected by the sex of the individual. For example, **sex-limited traits** are only

Reports that individuals who were XYY were prone to have violent tendencies were used as the basis of a series of fictional books and television programmes about 'The XYY Man'.

expressed in one sex, either female or male, but not both. An example of such a trait would be the production of milk in mammals.

However, some genetic patterns are said to be **sex-influenced**. Here, the sex of the individual may influence whether the phenotype in question is seen. For example, in sheep, some breeds have horns while others do not. If a heterozygous individual is bred from a cross of two such breeds it will have horns if it is male but will not have horns if it is female. Therefore the production of horns is influenced by the sex of the individual, but in the pure breeds both sexes may have horns and therefore the growth of horns is not exclusive to one sex. It is probable that the presence or absence of sex-related hormones is having an influence here.

Epistasis

> Epistasis may lead to odd ratios of offspring. Ratios of 9 : 7 are common, but others include 9 : 3 : 4, 13 : 3 or 15 : 1. Note they are all variations of 9 : 3 : 3 : 1 and all add up to 16.

In Mendelian inheritance Mendel was fortunate to have a situation where one gene led to the appearance of one phenotype. However, such simplicity is not always seen. For example, in a biochemical pathway the generation of a resultant product will be affected by the presence of all the enzymes in that pathway, which will in turn be affected by the presence of the required genes encoding those enzymes. Therefore, there is commonly interaction amongst genes to produce one phenotype, a phenomenon known as **epistasis**. This name comes from the Greek *epi* and *stasis*, meaning standing upon. A good example of such genetics is the production of cyanide in clover plants. This basically relies on the presence of two enzymes, one for the production of a metabolic intermediate and one for the conversion of that intermediate into cyanide. Plants that are able to make cyanide must have both enzymes, and therefore both genes. Plants that are unable to produce cyanide may be lacking in either gene, or in fact both genes.

Mutation

One of the obvious ways in which the inheritance pattern may not follow the rules laid down by Mendel is if there is an alteration within the DNA, and therefore a change in the product which the DNA codes for. Such **mutations**, if they take place within a section not important to the encoding of anything, will almost certainly have no effect on the individual or their offspring. However, mutations may cause the alteration of a gene product's activity, either impairing it or obliterating it, or may alter the expression pattern of the product. A mutation in the **promoter** sequence of a gene may stop the production of a protein which is normally produced, or alternatively, start the production of a protein from a normally quiescent gene. Such activity of **proto-oncogenes** contributes to the onset of cancer in many cases.

Mutations may simply be the alteration of a single base within the DNA, such an alteration being referred to as a **point mutation**.

Alternatively, larger stretches may have an **insertion, deletion** or **inversion**, the latter being where a stretch of DNA has been removed and reinserted in the same place but in the opposite orientation. If such insertion or deletion mutations alter the gene by a length of DNA bases that is not divisible by three, for example by removing or inserting only one or two bases, then all the subsequent codons read from that point on will be wrong and, therefore, through what might seem only slight alterations of the gene sequence there might be catastrophic alterations to the final protein product. Such an alteration is known as a **frame-shift mutation**.

Point mutations may result in **silent mutations**, where no alteration of the protein sequence is seen; for example, arginine may be coded for by the codons AGA or AGG. Therefore, if the original sequence was AGA but the last base is mutated from an A to a G, the new codon reads AGG and arginine will still be inserted into the protein and therefore no phenotype will be seen. Alternatively, if a new amino acid is coded for as a result of a point mutation, such an event is termed a **mis-sense mutation**. Such an event might be seen as having little or no effect on the resulting protein if that amino acid is in a relatively unimportant part of that protein, such as an external loop structure. However, if such changes take place within the active site of the protein, or influence the control of the protein, such a single base change could have a major effect on the protein's function.

On the other hand, if a UAU sequence, normally coding for a tyrosine, is altered to a UAG sequence, the latter is a stop codon. Therefore, when this RNA is being processed, instead of a tyrosine being added to the polypeptide and protein synthesis continuing, the sequence will read a stop, protein synthesis will cease and a **truncated protein** will result. Such a mutation is known as a **nonsense mutation**.

Suggested further reading

Hartl, D.L. and Orel, V. (1992). What did Gregor Mendel think he discovered? *Genetics*, **131**, 245.

Olby, R.C. (1966). *Origins of Mendelism*. Constable.

Orel, V. (1996). *Gregor Mendel: The First Geneticist*. Oxford University Press.

Peters, J.A. (1959). *Classic Papers in Genetics*. Prentice Hall.

Stern, C. and Sherwood, E. (1966). *The Origins of Genetics: A Mendel Source Book*. W.H. Freeman.

Todd, N.B. (1977). Cats and commerce. *Scientific American*, **237**, 100–107.

World Wide Web sites of interest

An interesting WWW page about Mendel can be found at:
http://www.netspace.org/MendelWeb/

Johann Gregor Mendel (1822–1884) Photo Archive:
http://www.open.cz/project/tourist/person/photo.htm

Self-assessment questions

1. If two F_1 plants with the genotype of Tt were bred together what is the ratio of the phenotypes in the F_2 generation, assuming Mendelian inheritance?
2. In what form are digenic inheritance patterns usually represented?
3. What is the common ratio seen with digenic inheritance, assuming Mendelian inheritance.
4. Why are carnation flowers which are heterozygous (Rr) pink and not the same as either parent if they were bred from red and white pure-breeding individuals?
5. If you breed Manx cats why are no homozygous MM individuals born?
6. How do human females inherit genes from the Y chromosome?
7. Genetically speaking, what is Turner's syndrome?
8. What is a frame-shift mutation?
9. What is a nonsense mutation?

Key Concepts and Facts

Gregor Mendel's Findings
- Mendel studied the inheritance mainly in peas but later worked on other species.

- Mendel chose seven characteristics to study, starting with pure-breeding plants.

- Mendel noted the characteristics of both the F_1 and F_2 generations.

- Alleles that always feature in the phenotype are referred to as dominant. Alleles that appear to get 'lost' and are dominated are referred to as being recessive.

- The F_2 generation gives a ratio of $3:1$ if one gene is studied.

- Digenic ratios are $9:3:3:1$.

- Digenic inheritance is often represented in the form of a Punnett square.

- Mendel's rules state briefly that alleles separate on meiosis and that this separation is independent of that of other alleles.

Exceptions to the Rules
- Many reasons lead to the alteration of simple Mendelian inheritance patterns.

- Incomplete dominance leads to a mixture of characteristics.

- Co-dominance leads to the appearance of both characteristics.

- Some allele combinations may be lethal.

- There may be many alleles for a particular characteristic.

- Genes may be carried by sex chromosomes and are therefore referred to as being sex-linked.

- The expression of genes may be sex-influenced.

- Mutations may have a profound effect on the phenotype.

- Metabolic pathways need the expression of more than one gene and therefore genes are seen to interact, a phenomenon referred to as epistasis.

Part Two
Techniques Used in Molecular Genetics

Chapter 9
Mapping of genes

Learning objectives

After studying this chapter you should confidently be able to:

Outline the process of recombination.

Explain what a linkage map is.

Describe the techniques used to obtain a gene map in pro-karyotes.

Describe the techniques used for mapping genes in yeast.

Define chromosome walking.

Outline gene mapping in humans.

In Part One we have discussed the structure of DNA and genes, and we have seen that genes are basically stretches of DNA where the information is encoded by the order of the bases along the DNA molecule. We have also seen that the DNA is arranged in chromosomes, or plasmids, etc., but one length of DNA will comprise several genes, and in many cases several thousand genes. Therefore, these genes which exist on the same length of DNA are said to be **linked**. If we inherit one chromosome, we would expect to inherit all the genes on that chromosome and for this to always be the case. However, this is not true, as chromosomes can undergo a process known as **recombination**, where lengths of DNA can break and recombine in a different order – so-called **crossovers**. This process was studied by Morgan at the start of the twentieth century, and by 1910 microscopic evidence was produced to support the hypothesis. This is very relevant to today's molecular geneticist as it is often important to find out where in the genome a particular gene is, on which chromosome and where on that chromosome it resides. Recombination can help greatly here. Also, this can be of particular importance in diseases where alterations of chromosomes such as deletions have occurred. Such information can also be used to clone genes by so-called **positional cloning** or **map-based cloning**.

Recombination

Recombination can be separated into three main types:

- Homologous recombination, or generalized recombination. This takes place between two sequences that are extensively homologous.
- Site-specific recombination. This takes place between sequences that have short stretches of homology.
- Non-homologous recombination or illegitimate recombination. This takes place between sequences which show no homology.

Mechanism of homologous recombination

Homologous recombination, or generalized recombination, may take place between two sequences in which the sequences are either the same or at least extremely similar. But how does this happen? One of the main proposals towards finding a mechanism was put forward by Robin Holliday, and this led to the scheme shown in Figure 9.1.

In this scheme there are several steps:

- The homologous DNA strands align.
- Cleavage points in single strands (known as nicks) are made in each of the DNA molecules.
- The strands displace to the opposite DNA.
- Ligation takes place, covalently linking to two DNAs. This results in a stable heteroduplex, known as a Holliday structure.

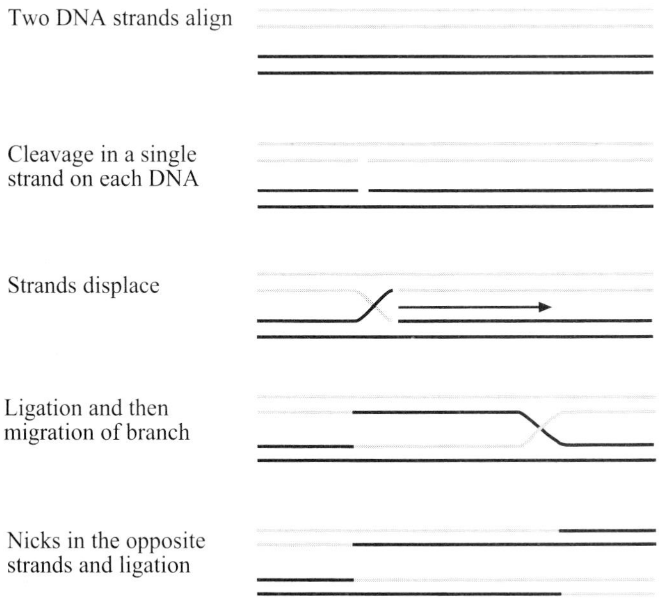

Two DNA strands align

Cleavage in a single strand on each DNA

Strands displace

Ligation and then migration of branch

Nicks in the opposite strands and ligation

Figure 9.1 *Mechanism of homologous recombination*

- The branch point migrates. Don't forget that the sequences are the same along this stretch of DNA and therefore the bases can swap over.
- The DNA is again cleaved and new DNA molecules are formed.

It is easier to understand the result of Figure 9.1 if Figure 9.2 is also referred to. Here the heteroduplex is redrawn, having introduced a twist. Strand breakage can then take place in two ways. If the opposite strand is cleaved from that originally cleaved in the first step, then the result is as shown in Figure 9.1 and Figure 9.2b. Here, the ends of the DNA molecules have been exchanged – a rather large change in the DNA. However, if the same strands are cleaved, then the result is as shown in Figure 9.2a. Here the changes are relatively minor.

Modifications to this scheme have been proposed. For example, the Meselson–Radding model, where the process is initiated by cleavage in only one strand and not both. It is suggested by this model that one strand 'invades' the other, the mechanism involving

> **Thomas Hunt Morgan**, born in 1866, studied at the University of Kentucky and Johns Hopkins University, although later much of his work was carried out at Columbia University, New York. In 1933 he was awarded the Nobel prize.

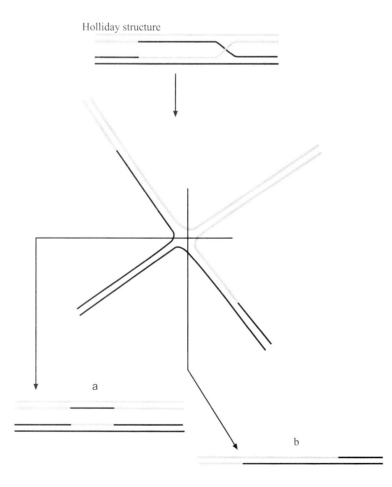

Holliday structure

Figure 9.2 *The Holliday structure may be redrawn in the chi form. This involves a twisting of the structure, but once redrawn it is easier to understand how the result shown in Figure 9.1 can be achieved or, alternatively, how a different result can be obtained, depending on which strands are broken in the second cleavage step*

what is referred to as a D-loop (or displacement loop). Similar models have been proposed by Hotchkiss, but here the loop is extended by replication of the DNA.

The role of recombination in nature

Recombination may take place between chromosomes and therefore, in eukaryotes, parental genes may effectively become merged. Recombination is also important in the integration of DNA into another DNA molecule, and also in the excision of DNA from a DNA molecule. In the life cycle of bacteriophages, for example, we see the integration of DNA into the genome. Lastly, in Chapter 4 we discussed transposons, and again their movement in a genome relies on recombination.

Recombination and mapping

If genes are located on the same chromosome then, when that chromosome is inherited by the next generation, it would be expected that both those genes would be passed on. These genes are said to be **linked**. Mendel stated in his principle of independent assortment that segregation of the members of any pair of alleles is independent of the segregation of the other pairs in the formation of the reproductive cells. Clearly, if genes are linked, physically, on the same chromosome this principle cannot be upheld.

In early experiments by Morgan, using *Drosophila,* he showed that, although the characteristics which he was studying were linked, the linkage was incomplete. Some new combinations of the characteristics were also observed. These new combinations were a result of a recombination event, which effectively 'unlinks' the genes. However, it has also been shown that the further apart the genes are on the chromosome, the more likely it is that a recombination event will take place (Figure 9.3). Therefore, by studying the frequency of the recombinations (or crossovers), a measure of the distance apart of the genes can be obtained, and therefore a **linkage map** or **chromosome map** may be drawn. Such maps were suggested by one of Morgan's students, Sturtevant, in 1913. Genes are assigned a segment of the chromosome called a **locus** (Figure 9.4).

Figure 9.3   *Three genes (a, b and c) that are linked. Recombination events between the genes would unlink them. Such recombinations, or crossovers, are much more likely between a and b than between a and c or b and c. These frequencies of recombination can be used to determine the spacings of the genes on the chromosome*

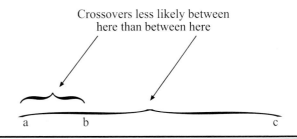

Crossovers less likely between here than between here

a   b   c

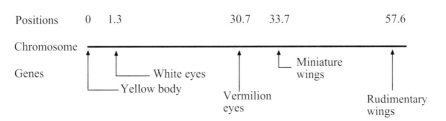

Figure 9.4   *Gene map of the X chromosome of* Drosophila, *as determined for five genes by Sturtevant*

The distance between genes in a map is given in **map units**. The frequency of recombination is given in per cent, and 1 map unit is equivalent to 1% recombination. One map unit is also called a **centimorgan** (cM). In reality, 1 map unit represents the length of chromosome in which one recombination event takes place per 50 cells undergoing meiosis.

However, there are one or two precautions necessary. If two genes are being studied in linkage experiments, and two recombination events take place between them, a so-called double crossover, then no alteration of the chromosome will be detected. Recombinations outside the regions between the two genes will also go undetected.

Recombination frequencies can be different in different sexes, and this can lead to different linkage maps being drawn up from different sexes of the same species. Also, some areas of the chromosome are more likely to undergo recombination than others, for example in regions of heterochromatin which forms dense structures during the interphase stage of meiosis.

> The minimum recombination frequency obtainable is 0%. The highest frequency is 50%. This is equivalent to two genes which assort independently.

How are maps derived in the laboratory?

Early genetic maps drawn up by Morgan and his students relied on the crossing of individuals showing certain characteristics and then studying the offspring, in the same way as Mendel carried out his experiments. With species that multiply and breed quickly this is a valid option, but it is more difficult for species with long breeding periods or where dictated breeding is impossible, as in humans.

Mapping in bacteria

The mapping of genes in bacteria is carried out using one of three techniques, but they are all based on the same principle. The steps that need to take place are as outlined below:

- Two strains of bacteria are needed. The donor strain should contain wild-type copies of the genes of interest. The recipient strain should contain mutated versions of these genes.
- Gene transfer from donor to recipient cells. This might involve the transfer of all or part of the DNA.

- Recombination. This might be a double recombination with the resultant removal and degradation of the original copies of the genes in the recipient.
- Selection. Using selective growth media recipient cells which contain only the unmutated genes from the donor will survive to be analysed.

The three main techniques for mapping basically differ in their methods of gene transfer. This might be achieved by:

- Conjugation
- Transduction
- Transformation.

Conjugation

Bacteria such as *E. coli* can exchange DNA between cells by a process known as **conjugation** (see Figure 9.5). This process is controlled by a plasmid known as the F plasmid, which in *E. coli* is 95 kb. The plasmid encodes several genes including those which are involved in the formation of the pilus, the tube through which the DNA passes in the transfer process.

The plasmid itself transfers from the donor cell (so-called F$^+$) to the F$^-$ recipient cell, through the pilus, but a copy is left behind, ensuring that the donor remains F$^+$. Importantly, however, mechanisms exist which enable some of the other *E. coli* DNA to be transferred too. This might take place by chance, or be more directed after integration of the F plasmid into the cell's DNA.

How does this help us map genes? The process of conjugation proceeds by transfer of the linear DNA through the pilus into the recipient. All the DNA does not appear in the recipient together, rather it is fed in like a length of string. Therefore, some genes arrive before others, that is gene transfer is sequential. Elie Wollman and François Jacob devised a method of interrupted conjugation. Conjugation was allowed to proceed for a set length of time and then the pilus disrupted by agitation. Only the genes that are transferred early are therefore able to be found in the recipient cells, and altering the length of time conjugation is allowed to proceed will enable the order of transfer of the genes to be determined. As some of the *E. coli* DNA is able to be transferred as well as the F plasmid itself, then the *E. coli* genome may be

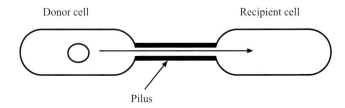

Figure 9.5 *The process of conjugation*

mapped by such methods. However, this technique can only be used in bacteria which undergo conjugation.

Transformation and transduction

DNA can also be transferred from one individual bacterium to another by either **transduction** or **transformation**. In the latter, fragments of DNA, sometimes referred to as naked DNA, are taken up by the recipient cells. Certain species of bacteria are more likely to do this than others. For example, *Bacillus* species take up DNA relatively easily but it is quite hard to achieve with *E. coli*. With transduction the uptake of the DNA is mediated by a bacteriophage. The transduction phage P22 is able to package approximately 40 kb of DNA. There is a low but significant chance that the phage will package a fragment of the cell's genomic DNA instead of copies of its own genome. Therefore, these new phages will bind to and inject into the recipient cells copies of the host cell's genes, and gene transfer has occurred. The introduced DNA fragment will undergo recombination with the recipient genome and become integrated.

In both transduction and transformation the host genome may be transferred to a recipient cell. Therefore new genes which code for recognizable characteristics may be introduced. Commonly, as with conjugation, a wild-type gene may be introduced into a mutated cell. How does this help in mapping? If the fragments of host DNA contain two genes which are relatively close together (less than 40 kb in the case of transduction due to the packing restraint of the phage), then the new characteristics can be looked for in the recipient cells. If both are found together, then the genes are mapped close together. An extension of the technique involves looking for the introduction of perhaps three genes and, using the frequencies of the introduction of the characteristics, enables their order to be determined and a map drawn.

Mapping in yeast

Mapping is not confined to prokaryotes. Yeast are often used as a model eukaryotic system and mapping experiments are common. Certain strains of yeast are haploid which will aid in the interpretation of mapping experiments. In addition, during their life cycle yeast gamete cells will fuse to form a zygote which will then subsequently divide by meiosis, resulting in a **tetrad** containing four cells, referred to as an **ascospore**. These ascospores are contained in a structure called the **ascus**. The ascus will burst, releasing the ascospores which can divide by mitosis (Figure 9.6).

As with bacterial cells, certain characteristics may be looked for in yeast; for example, a dependence on certain ingredients of the growth medium such as alanine or leucine. Alternatively, they may be resistant to an additive to the growth medium such as copper or cycloheximide.

Certain bacterial cells such as *E. coli* do not readily take up DNA. However, using certain treatments their DNA uptake can be increased. Such cells are said to be competent.

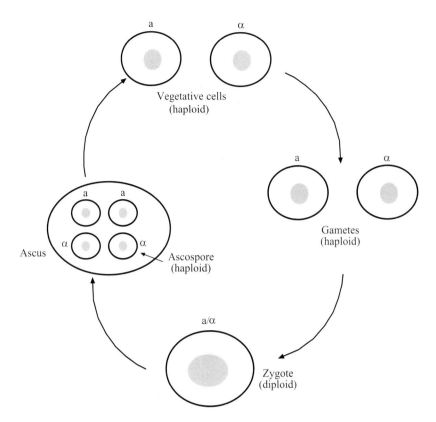

Figure 9.6 *Simplified scheme of the life cycle of yeast (*Saccharomyces cerevisiae*). This strain has haploid vegetative cells which differentiate to haploid gametes. The zygote is therefore diploid, but meiosis gives rise to haploid ascospores. Bursting of the ascus and mitosis give rise once again to haploid vegetative cells*

In a mapping experiment, strains of the opposite mating type are used, one of which contains the gene of interest, perhaps a wild-type gene, and the other a mutant for this gene. After mixing the cells, the resulting progeny may be screened for the presence of the gene. The cells may be screened in two ways:

- Random spore analysis: A sample of the ascospores is spread on agar. Replicate plates are used which contain the required growth additive or not. The frequency of the cells which contain the transferred gene can therefore be calculated.

- Tetrad analysis: Individual asci (plural of ascus) can be separated, broken open and the ascospores grown on agar.

As with bacterial cells, two or more genes may be studied to determine the frequency of transfer to the progeny. The frequencies will once again depend on the frequency of recombinations or crossovers, and therefore an approximate map may be drawn up by random spore analysis. Combinations of the characteristics may be more accurately determined by tetrad analysis. If two parental characteristics are of interest, and the parents are therefore x^+z^+ and x^-z^-, the resulting tetrads may contain the following combinations:

- Ascospores may contain only the parental gene combinations, called the parental ditype (PD). Genotypes will be x^+z^+ or x^-z^-.
- Ascospores may contain the non-parental combinations, that is x^+z^- or x^-z^+. There will be two of each. This is referred to as the non-parental ditype (NPD).
- Ascospores may contain all possible combinations. This is a tetratype (TT), the four combinations of genes being: x^+z^+, x^+z^-, x^-z^+, x^-z^-.

Once again, by calculation of the frequencies of the combinations, the distances between the genes may be estimated and a genetic map drawn.

Chromosome walking

If two genes are thought to be extremely close together, and the position of one is known, then the second can be found by **chromosome walking**. Here, two gene libraries are needed (see Chapter 11). A probe containing the sequence of the first gene is used to hybridize to the DNA in one library and then the resulting clones obtained are used to probe the second library. By alternating the use of the libraries, because hybridization will only take place if the sequences overlap, it is possible to 'walk' down the DNA. However, this is a very lengthy procedure and only short lengths of DNA can be studied by this method. The longest distance able to be analysed by this method is probably of the order of only 250 kb. However, probably the greatest success of this technique is the finding of the gene responsible for cystic fibrosis. This is a single gene that encodes a protein known as **cystic fibrosis transmembrane regulator** (CFTR) which functions as a chloride channel in the epithelial cells.

Mapping in humans

Mapping in humans is particularly problematical, as breeding experiments are clearly not possible. However, mapping is possible and, in fact, the Human Genome Project will relatively soon not only map the entire human genome but also have a representative sequence for the genome too.

One useful method is to study the human genome, or any other genome, using restriction endonucleases. Because restriction endonucleases only cleave the DNA at very specific sequences, if sequence alternations are introduced to the genome, then new restriction endonuclease cleavage sites may be introduced, or alternatively removed. Therefore it is possible to use these endonucleases to

Because the gene that causes cystic fibrosis has now been identified, there is hope that gene therapy may one day give a lasting cure for the disease. This is further discussed in Chapter 14.

look for differences between individuals' genomes. Differences discovered between individuals using endonucleases are known as **restriction fragment length polymorphisms** (RFLPs). Disease states can be particularly useful here, as a phenotype is known and a comparison with the normal genome carried out.

Many other methods of mapping large genomes are available to the modern molecular geneticist – too many to be discussed here. Such methods include the use of marker sequences and *in situ* **hybridization**; for more detail the reader is referred to the suggested further reading list below.

Suggested further reading

Brown, T.A. (1998). *Genetics: A Molecular Approach*, 3rd edn. Chapman and Hall. (Chapters 18 and 19 in particular.)

Eggleston, A.K. and West, S.C. (1996). Exchanging partners: recombination in *E. coli. Trends in Genetics*, **12**, 20–26.

Hartl, D.L. (1996). *Essential Genetics*. Jones and Bartlett. (Chapter 4 in particular.)

Hartl, D.L. and Jones, E.W. (1998). *Genetics: Principles and Analysis*, 4th edn. Jones and Bartlett. (Chapter 4 in particular.)

Holliday, R. (1964). A mechanism for gene conversion in fungi. *Genetical Research*, **5**, 282–304.

Primrose, S.B. (1998). *Principles of Genome Analysis*, 2nd edn. Blackwell Science. (Chapter 4 in particular for more in-depth methods of genome mapping.)

White, R. and Lalouel, J.M. (1988). Chromosome mapping with DNA markers. *Scientific American*, **258**, 40.

Self-assessment questions

1. What feature distinguishes homologous recombination from non-homologous recombination?
2. Who put forward a scheme to explain the mechanism of recombination and now has one of the structures postulated named after them?
3. What are the units of the genetic map?
4. List three methods of gene transfer in bacteria.
5. Name the method used to find the gene responsible for cystic fibrosis.
6. Why are Mendel's rules relevant to gene mapping?
7. What name is given to the segment on a chromosome where a gene is said to reside?
8. What is the name of the plasmid that controls bacterial conjugation?
9. Which method of gene transfer in bacteria relies on a phage?

Key Concepts and Facts

Recombination

- Recombination allows the exchange of genetic material.

- Recombination may take place between homologous regions of DNA or between sequences which are not related.

- The mechanism of recombination involves strand cleavage and the formation of a Holliday structure.

- Recombination frequency can be used to map genes.

- Recombination is used by many organisms in nature.

Mapping

- The frequency of recombination can be converted to map units or centimorgans to measure distances between genes.

- Mapping in bacteria is achieved by studying gene transfer.

- Gene transfer in bacteria may be achieved by conjugation, transformation or transduction.

- Mapping in yeast can be carried out using random spore analysis or tetrad analysis.

- A gene which is relatively close to another may be found by chromosome walking.

- Many methods are available to map human genes but breeding is not possible.

Chapter 10
Gel electrophoresis and blotting

Learning objectives

After studying this chapter you should confidently be able to:

Outline what information may be sought about a sample of DNA or RNA.

Describe the electrophoresis of a DNA/RNA sample.

Outline how one might assess the purity of a sample of nucleic acid.

Describe the methods of studying DNA by Southern analysis.

Describe the methods of studying RNA by Northern analysis.

One of the challenges of molecular genetics is to isolate segments of DNA and to assign to them a sequence and therefore a possible function. Similarly with RNA, its isolation and identification are often crucial towards the understanding of the molecular mechanisms occurring within a cell. Therefore this chapter will concentrate on the analysis of the DNA or RNA which has been isolated. Questions commonly being asked are:

- How pure is my sample?
- How much DNA/RNA do I have?
- What is the size of the fragment?
- Where does it occur or when is it expressed?

Here some, but not all, of the techniques which can be used to attempt to answer these questions will be described.

Electrophoresis

Often the researcher will need to separate the fractions of DNA/RNA that have been isolated and attempt to identify what is there. To do this, a common technique is to separate samples through a gel material in the presence of an electric field, a process known as **electrophoresis**. This is one of the techniques most commonly used by the molecular geneticist. Electrophoresis is defined as the movement of charged molecules in an electric field. This is very applicable here because DNA is negatively charged. The electrophoresis is carried out using a gel, and in many cases this gel is made from **agarose**. The gel, when formed, will contain a network of small pores, through which the migrating molecules must pass. Therefore, the smaller the molecules, the easier it is for them to travel and the further they will go. The larger molecules are retarded and therefore the DNA will separate according to its size. It should be noted that very large molecules might be retained to such an extent that no migration takes place at all, and they will remain at the top of the gel. In practice, the researcher simply has to dissolve the correct amount of agarose in an appropriate buffer, pour this into a casing chamber and allow the gel to set. A comb is inserted into the setting gel which, when removed, leaves small wells in the gel, into which the sample can be placed (see Figure 10.1). Alternatively, gels may be made using **polyacrylamide**, which is used routinely if separation of proteins is being sought.

Once the gel has been cast, the samples are mixed with a charged dye, usually bromophenol blue, which is so small that it will

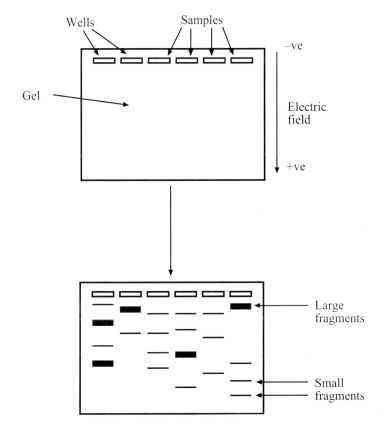

Figure 10.1 *Agarose gel electrophoresis. A schematic diagram of a gel before and after the application of the electric field*

Figure 10.2 *Photograph of a real gel on which DNA has been analysed. Note that the DNA shows as a bright band on a dark background, the opposite to most protein gels. (Kindly supplied by Dr Radhika Desikan, UWE)*

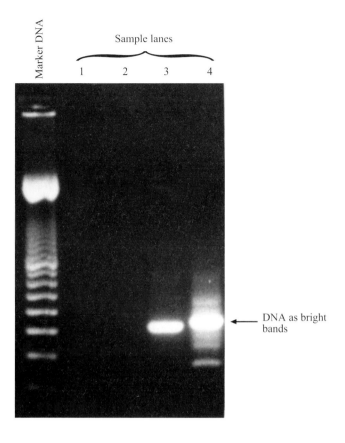

Intercalating dyes bind to the DNA by adopting a position between the bases.

migrate faster than any DNA molecules and therefore act as an indicator of how far the smallest DNA has run through the gel. Also, DNA molecules of known sizes are analysed alongside the unknown samples to give an indication of the size of the sample DNAs (see Figure 10.2).

The DNA on the gel is visualized by either the inclusion in the gel of an **intercalating dye**, ethidium bromide, or by soaking the gel in the dye after it has run. The gel is then placed on a transilluminating light box, which emits UV light. Any ethidium bromide which is associated with DNA will fluoresce and therefore the DNA will be seen as a bright band on a dark background. It is then simply a case of photographing the results. For convenience, most researchers use a Polaroid (instant) camera so that the results may be very rapidly recorded and acted upon. An example of such a gel analysis is shown in Figure 10.2.

Purity and concentration of nucleotides

Before many molecular genetics experiments can be performed, it is important to assess both the purity and the quantity (or concentration) of the DNA or RNA being used. Typically this

RNA or DNA may have been isolated from tissues or cells and is then used for gel electrophoresis or cloning, and may therefore be contaminated with other nucleotides, proteins or lipids.

Spectroscopy

Like many biological materials, nucleotides such as DNA and RNA have a characteristic light absorbance pattern, and this can be used as a measure of both the purity and concentration. Typically, a small quantity of the test material is diluted and put into a cuvette, which is placed in a **spectrophotometer**. The absorbance of light is then measured in the UV part of the spectrum. Either a **spectrum** is recorded between 200 nm and 300 nm, as shown in Figure 10.3, or the absorbance at 260 nm and 280 nm is recorded separately. DNA and RNA both absorb light at 260 nm, while proteins have a strong absorbance at 280 nm. This can be used as an indication of the purity of the sample. Furthermore, by determining the 260/280 ratio, an indication of whether the material is primarily DNA or RNA is obtained: DNA has a ratio of 1.8, while RNA has a ratio of 2 or above. Ratios of less than 1.8 indicate contamination, usually by either protein or the residues of phenol used in the extraction procedures.

Also, as for other biological materials, the absorbance of the light at 260 nm is directly proportional to the amount of material present. This extinction coefficient can then be used to calculate the quantity of the material in the sample.

> The extinction coefficient of DNA is such that an absorbance of 1 corresponds to 50 μg per ml of double-stranded DNA.

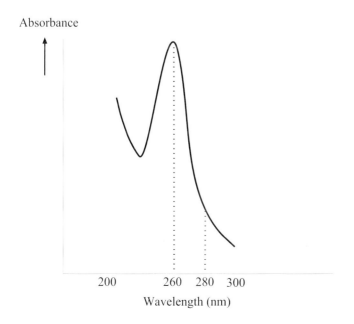

Absorbance

Wavelength (nm)

Figure 10.3 *Typical spectrum of a sample of DNA. Light absorbance was measured between 200 nm and 300 nm*

Figure 10.4 *Diagram of an RNA gel used to assess the purity of the sample. A, DNA shows as a bright band at the top of the gel; B, broken-down RNA smears towards the bottom of the gel; C, good total RNA also shows that the rRNA is still intact, indicating that the RNA has not been broken down*

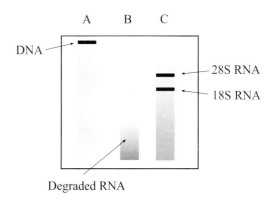

Gel electrophoresis

Agarose gel electrophoresis can also be used as a measure of the purity of samples, and this is particularly useful when RNA is being used. RNA is notoriously unstable, and therefore molecular geneticists regularly analyse isolated RNA by gel electrophoresis to assess not only the purity but also the integrity of the sample. A typical gel is shown in Figure 10.4. As can be seen, on an RNA gel, DNA will show as a bright band near the top of the gel, while broken down RNA will show as a bright smear towards the bottom of the gel. Good usable total cellular RNA will show as a bright smear which spans the gel but will also show brighter bands indicating that rRNA in the sample has not been broken down.

Analysis by blotting

Southern blotting

A question commonly asked is, does the DNA from a genome or isolated sample contain the stretch of DNA, perhaps a gene, that the researcher is interested in? One way of answering such a question is by Southern analysis, commonly referred to as Southern transfer or Southern blotting. This technique was reported in 1975 by Professor E.M. Southern. Other techniques for dealing with RNA and protein were subsequently developed and dubbed with the names Northern and Western blotting, respectively.

In Southern blotting, the sample of DNA fragments of interest is separated by gel electrophoresis and then 'blotted' or transferred on to a sheet of nitrocellulose or equivalent. The blotting apparatus is, in fact, very simple, as depicted in Figure 10.5.

The membrane is simply placed on the gel and the buffer soaks through, carrying the DNA with it. The buffer is continuously supplied by a wick (of filter paper) from a reservoir, and continuously absorbed on the other side of the membrane by a pile of paper towels held under a weight. As the DNA meets the nitrocellulose it binds and therefore the pattern of DNA on the

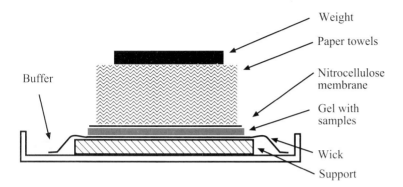

Buffer

Weight

Paper towels

Nitrocellulose membrane

Gel with samples

Wick

Support

Figure 10.5 *Diagram of the Southern transfer apparatus commonly used. Often this is created out of odds and ends from the laboratory, although expensive, complicated and very efficient alternatives are on the market*

membrane precisely matches that which was on the gel after separation. The gel is then fixed by UV light or heating and the membrane can then be used for analysis.

For analysis, the fact that DNA strands naturally hybridize together according to their sequence is made use of. To find a particular DNA sequence a probe is used which has the complementary sequence. The probe, under the correct conditions, will only hybridize or bind to the DNA on the membrane with the correct matching sequence. Therefore, out of all the bands on the membrane, perhaps only one or two will bind to the probe. How do you find where the probe is bound? The easiest way is to make the probe radioactive. This can be achieved in several ways depending on the nature of the probes used.

Probes may be synthesized chemically, creating a short oligo-nucleotide, as we shall see again in Chapter 12. Therefore radio-active nucleotides may be incorporated. However, such probes are usually very short and the longer the probe the better, giving better hybridization and much greater specificity, with less chance of the wrong result. Alternatively, probes may be created using the polymerase chain reaction (Chapter 12) and again there is a chance here to incorporate radioactive nucleotides. However, cloned DNA fragments also make good probes. Here, commonly a kinase is used to radiolabel one end of the probe, by the incorporation of a radioactive phosphate, but using this method only allows the incorporation of one radioactive atom per probe molecule. If nucleotide incorporation is used as an alternative, then radioactivity can be included every time that nucleotide (say an A) is added to the growing sequence. Therefore, the final signal is much greater.

In practice, once the probe has been made, the membrane is washed in the presence of the probe. Subsequent washes, of increasing **stringency**, remove the unbound or weakly bound probe, and then the membrane is sandwiched next to a photographic film and left for the desired time, depending on how much radioactivity is used. The film is simply processed to get the result. This process is known as **autoradiography**.

Many laboratories are now trying to reduce the amount of radioactivity used in various techniques, for obvious safety reasons. Nucleotide labels that are non-radioactive are available and work very well.

Figure 10.6 *Scheme to show the steps taken in Southern blotting*

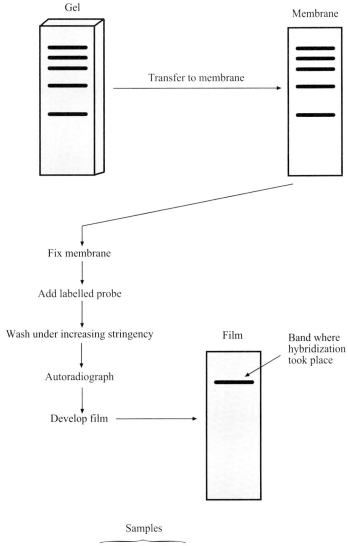

Figure 10.7 *Real results of a Southern blotting experiment. The dark bands show where hybridization of the probe with the DNA on the membrane took place. (Kindly supplied by Dr Radhika Desikan, UWE)*

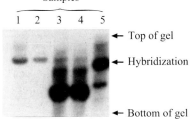

The steps of Southern blotting are sketched out in Figure 10.6, while a real result is shown in Figure 10.7.

Northern blotting

Northern analysis is very similar to Southern analysis, except here RNA is used and not DNA. The question commonly being asked when Northern analysis is employed is, does this cell express this gene under these conditions? Here we are looking for the mRNA transcript of the gene, and hence can then determine if the gene is being expressed or not. Commonly cells may be analysed under different conditions. For example, the researcher may like to know if a cytokine, such as tumour necrosis factor, switches on the expression of a certain gene, for example another cytokine. Here Northern analysis will be able to supply an answer.

Several warnings need to be given here. If no signal is found after Northern analysis it might not mean that the cell is not expressing the gene. It may be that the levels of expression are so low that Northern analysis is simply not sensitive enough. One way around this problem is to employ alternative techniques such as RT-PCR (see Chapter 12). Secondly, the finding of the mRNA for a gene does not necessarily mean that the mRNA is used and translated into protein. To be sure that the protein is being expressed in a cell other techniques such as Western blotting are needed, and commonly papers will report the use of both Northern and Western blotting to give a more complete picture.

Having been somewhat critical, however, Northern analysis is a very useful and powerful tool. Many papers have used it to report the induction of certain genes by other factors such as hormones, or to show which cells and tissues in an organism are expressing certain genes.

The experimental procedure is very similar to that depicted in Figure 10.6. The gel for the separation of the RNA commonly is different to that used to separate DNA, the gel here being a denaturing one including formamide, but the subsequent steps and the end result are similar. A real Northern analysis result can be seen in Figure 10.8.

The starting material for the Northern analysis need not be purified mRNA, and the total RNA from the cells may be used. This would of course include rRNA and tRNA. This works well if the mRNA of interest is relatively abundant. However, if the mRNA to be analysed is expressed at only a very low level, then purification of the mRNA fraction may be required before the gel is run and analysed.

One of the advantages of Northern analysis is that it is quantifiable. The darkness of the bands on the gel are related to the amount of mRNA present in the starting material. Therefore, it is possible to

> Stringency of hybridization refers to the conditions under which hybridization takes place. The hybridization of two stretches of DNA is influenced by salt concentrations and temperature, both of which are altered experimentally to ensure that only the correct hybridization takes place. At high stringency, only the complementary strands will hybridize, but under low stringency, DNA strands which are less complementary can still hybridize, often leading to incorrect and misleading results.

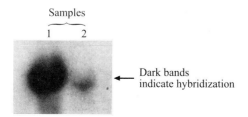

Samples

1   2

← Dark bands indicate hybridization

Figure 10.8 *Real results of a Northern analysis experiment. (Kindly supplied by Dr Radhika Desikan, UWE)*

measure levels of expression, and with modern densitometer scanners it is relatively easy to translate the darkness of the bands on a film into real numbers which can be compared. Clearly, however, realistic comparisons can only be made if the two samples are run on the same gel and exposed on the same film, as the exposure time of the film is critical to the final analysis.

Suggested further reading

Alvine, J.C., Kemp, D.J., Parker, B.A., Renart, J., Stark, G.R. and Wahl, G.M. (1979). Detection of specific RNAs or specific fragments of DNA by fractionation in gels and transfer to diazobenzyloxymethyl paper. *Methods in Enzymology*, **68**, 220–242. (Early paper on Northern blotting.)

Conner, B.J., Reyes, A.A., Morin, C., Itakura, K., Teplitz, R. and Wallace, R. (1983). Detection of sickle cell β^s-globin allele by hybridisation with synthetic oligonucleotides. *Proceedings of the National Academy of Sciences, USA*, **80**, 278–282.

Desikan, R., Reynolds, A., Hancock, J.T. and Neill, S.J. (1998). Harpin and hydrogen peroxide both initiate programmed cell death but have differential effects on defence gene expression in *Arabidopsis* suspension cultures. *Biochemical Journal*, **330**, 115–120. (An example where Northern analysis has been used.)

Southern, E.M. (1975). Detection of specific sequences among DNA fragments separated by gel electrophoresis. *Journal of Molecular Biology*, **98**, 503–507. (Original paper on Southern blotting.)

Thomas, P.S. (1980). Hybridisation of denatured RNA and small DNA fragments transferred to nitrocellulose. *Proceedings of the National Academy of Sciences, USA*, **77**, 5201–5205. (Refinement of the Northern technique.)

Self-assessment questions

1. What is the difference between Southern and Northern analysis?
2. What is Western analysis used for?
3. Name one type of material that can be used to bind to DNA in a Southern analysis.
4. Name two methods that could be used to assess the purity of an RNA sample.
5. What are gels for DNA analysis commonly made with?
6. Once a probe has been allowed to hybridize to a DNA sample after transfer to a membrane, how is the presence of the probe analysed?
7. In gel electrophoresis the DNA separates according to size. Where on the gel are the largest DNA fragments and where are the smallest?
8. Define electrophoresis.

Key Concepts and Facts

Background Facts
- A common aim in molecular genetics is to analyse DNA and RNA samples.

- DNA and RNA can be separated by electrophoresis.

- DNA and RNA can be visualized by the use of dyes such as ethidium bromide.

- The purity of DNA and RNA can be assessed by spectroscopy and by electrophoresis.

Analysis by Blotting
- Southern analysis was named after the person who reported the technique. Northern and Western analysis were subsequently developed.

- Southern analysis is used for the study of DNA.

- Northern analysis is used for the study of RNA.

- Western analysis is used for the study of proteins.

- Samples are separated by electrophoresis and then transferred to a membrane for further analysis.

- Analysis of the presence of DNA/RNA is carried out using DNA probes.

- Commonly, probes are made radioactive and their presence sought by autoradiography.

Chapter 11
Gene cloning and gene libraries

Learning objectives

After studying this chapter you should confidently be able to:

Describe the steps needed to be taken in gene cloning.

Describe two methods of DNA extraction.

Outline the cutting of DNA.

Explain how DNA is joined back together again.

Outline the characteristics of a good cloning vector.

Appreciate the use of plasmids as cloning vectors.

Appreciate the use of bacteriophages as cloning vectors.

Describe cosmids.

Describe the types of gene library and their uses.

One of the greatest advances made in molecular genetics is the ability to manipulate DNA, to remove sections, add sections and join bits together. Because it is now possible to take a length of DNA and join it to another length, commonly from another species, it is now possible to introduce genes into organisms either so that the functionality of that DNA may be studied, or to alter the characteristics of the organism itself. This latter point will be explored more in Chapter 14. However, here we will describe the cutting, joining and manipulation of DNA which has allowed this expansion of DNA technology.

Cloning

Gene cloning, otherwise referred to as **recombinant DNA technology** or **genetic engineering**, involves introduction of a DNA fragment into an organism so that a population of organisms is created with the same gene or genes present. The steps involved include:

1. Isolation of DNA fragment of interest

2. Introduce DNA fragment into vector by restriction cutting and ligation

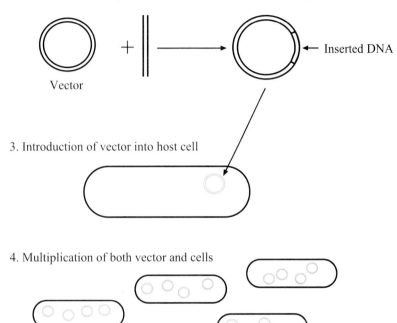

Vector

Inserted DNA

3. Introduction of vector into host cell

4. Multiplication of both vector and cells

Figure 11.1 *Schematic representation of the strategy used to clone a DNA fragment*

- The isolation of the length of DNA of interest.
- The introduction of this DNA into a second DNA molecule which will ease its introduction into the host organism. This second DNA is referred to as a **vector**. The vector and inserted DNA together are referred to as a recombinant DNA molecule.
- The introduction of the vector containing the DNA fragment back into a host organism.
- Multiplication of the vector within the host organism and cell division of the host organism, resulting in many cells all containing the new DNA.

These steps are represented schematically in Figure 11.1 and we will discuss some of the procedures and techniques required in turn.

Manipulation of DNA

DNA isolation

Often DNA needs to be isolated quickly, and with the minimum of effort. Several methods have been developed to achieve this. One of

Phenol has to be handled with extreme care, as it burns. Usually it is used in a fume hood with exposed skin covered.

the popular methods used is **phenol extraction**. Here, a cell extract is mixed with phenol or a phenol/chloroform mixture (1 : 1). The mixture is then centrifuged to separate the layers. Proteins are precipitated as a white mass at the interface which forms between the phenol at the bottom of the centrifuge tube and the aqueous layer which floats on top. The DNA and usually RNA will be dissolved in the aqueous layer which can be drawn off. To remove excessive levels of protein, sometimes treatment with a protease such as proteinase K or pronase is needed prior to extraction. To remove RNA, the DNA isolated can be treated with ribonuclease.

An alternative method of DNA purification can involve the use of an **anion exchange resin**. Here, the positively charged beads are used to attract and bind to the negatively charged nucleic acids which can be collected after the resins have been washed to remove unwanted material.

Ultracentrifugation

Centrifugation has commonly been used by biochemists for the separation and isolation of both cells and cellular material, and in this respect the isolation of DNA is little different. However, unlike whole cells which sediment relatively rapidly, DNA needs high centrifugal forces, of the order of several hundred thousand $\times \boldsymbol{g}$, and therefore isolation may require an ultracentrifuge. Such a machine was invented in 1924 by the Swede, **Svedberg**. Two main types of ultracentrifugation are commonly used:

- **Density gradient centrifugation**. Here a density gradient is set up inside the centrifuge tube, and the sample DNA will migrate to a point on the density gradient which matches its own density. Gradients are commonly formed by the centrifugation of **CsCl**. CsCl will be forced to the bottom of the tube by centrifugation, but will try to migrate back due to diffusion, and hence a gradient is formed. Typically this gradient may be from $1.6 \, \text{g cm}^{-3}$ CsCl to $1.8 \, \text{g cm}^{-3}$ CsCl. An example of an experiment can be seen in Figure 11.2.

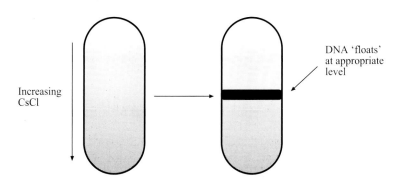

Figure 11.2 *Schematic representation of ultracentrifugation. A CsCl gradient is used to separate DNA, which 'floats' as a band at the appropriate density*

Increasing CsCl

DNA 'floats' at appropriate level

- **Velocity centrifugation.** Here it is the speed of migration through a dense solution which is important. The solution may be sucrose, which is also commonly used in the separation of subcellular organelles. The rate of migration is expressed as a sedimentation coefficient, or S value, where S is a Svedberg unit. In Part One we saw how ribosomal subunits were expressed as 60S etc., depending on their sedimentation coefficient. It is the same techniques that may be used with DNA.

> **Theodor Svedberg** was born in 1884 and died in 1971. He was a Swedish chemist who invented the first ultracentrifuge in 1924, for which he received the Nobel prize for Chemistry in 1926.

Cutting DNA

To manipulate DNA one of the fundamental techniques needed is to be able to cut the DNA at the desired position. This can be achieved by the use of a class of enzymes called **restriction endonucleases**, often referred to as **restriction enzymes**. They were so called because their function in cells is to cleave foreign DNA in prokaryotes, and so restrict the use of DNA within the foreign cell. They were discovered by Werner Arber, Hamilton Smith and Daniel Nathans in the late 1960s and now nearly one hundred have been purified. They are named in a systematic way, using:

1. A three letter abbreviation of the organism from which they were isolated.

2. A designation of the strain of that organism.

3. A roman numeral for the number of enzymes produced by those cells.

An example would be *Eco*RI, from *E. coli*.

Restriction enzymes fall into two groups. Some of the enzymes recognize a sequence of DNA and cut the DNA on both strands at the same place. These result in the DNA being cut with **blunt ends** (see Figure 11.3). Alternatively, some enzymes recognize the sequence on the DNA and cut either side of the centre of this sequence and therefore leave an overhang on each DNA, so-called **sticky ends**, as shown in Figure 11.3. Often the type of restriction enzyme used will be chosen because it leaves blunt or sticky ends, as this might aid in the next step of the procedure. For example, rejoining the DNA is often easier if sticky ends are present.

Because the exact cut sites in the DNA made by each restriction enzyme are known, computers can be used to predict if and where a gene may be cut by particular enzymes and specific enzymes chosen accordingly. If a gene is to be cloned into a new site, it would be unwise to choose a restriction enzyme which will cut the gene into several pieces. Commonly, DNA is cleaved completely by particular restriction enzymes and the fragments so generated analysed by electrophoresis to give what is referred to as a **restriction map**. Such a map will be characteristic of a particular length of DNA with a particular enzyme and, once known, can be used to identify DNA.

Figure 11.3 *Cuts made by restriction endonucleases. (1) Some enzymes leave blunt-ended DNA; (2) other enzymes leave sticky ends. Note that the cut sequences are palindromic*

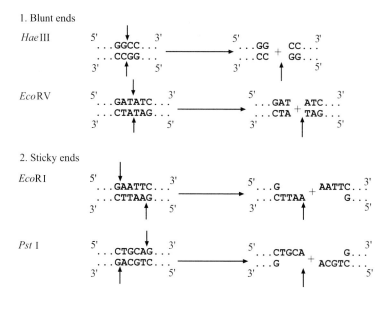

Figure 11.4 *Schematic representation of a restriction map. The lane on the left shows uncut DNA which runs as a band near the top of the gel. The lane on the right shows the fragments generated by total cleavage of the DNA by the restriction endonuclease chosen*

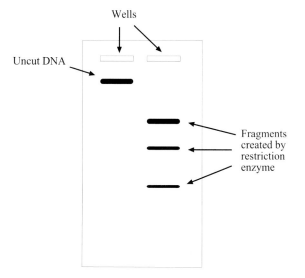

An example of a restriction map is schematically drawn in Figure 11.4.

Joining DNA back together

Once the DNA has been cut, commonly it needs to be joined to another DNA molecule, for example a **vector**. This process of joining DNA together is called **ligation** and is catalysed by a class of enzymes known as **ligases**. These enzymes were discovered in 1967 and catalyse the formation of a bond between the 3′-OH group on one DNA to the 5′-phosphate group of the other. It is an energy-dependent reaction and requires either ATP or NAD$^+$ depending on the enzyme.

Ligases will rejoin either blunt ends or sticky ends but the joining of sticky ends is more efficient. Sticky ends will, by nature, temporarily hybridize and stick together, giving the ligase an opportunity to catalyse the bond formation. However, blunt ends do not have this capacity and therefore it is much more of a chance reaction.

Cloning vectors

A vector is a DNA molecule which can replicate in a suitable host organism, and into which a fragment of DNA may be introduced. Vectors may need to have the following characteristics:

- Be easily introduced into the host organism. This is known as **transformation** using plasmids or **transfection** using phages.
- Have a site or sites which can be cleaved by a restriction endonuclease, where the DNA fragment can be introduced.
- Have a site of replication (replication origin) and can therefore replicate in the host organism.
- Be selectable in some way. Often this is because the vector also contains a gene which confers antibiotic resistance on the host organism.

A typical cloning strategy would be to isolate the vector, cleave the vector at the chosen restriction endonuclease site, and then mix the vector and the insert DNA fragment together in the presence of a ligase. It is hoped that the insert will be ligated into the vector at this chosen site, as shown in part 2 of Figure 11.1. However, there is also a high probability that the vector will simply be ligated back together again with no fragment of DNA inserted. This latter case would just yield the wild-type vector and be of no further use. Cloning strategies have therefore been developed to select for the vectors which have inserted DNA, as discussed briefly below.

Plasmids as vectors

Plasmids are commonly used as vectors. These contain an **origin of replication**, contain several restriction endonuclease cut sites which can be used for insertion of the 'new' DNA, and commonly carry genes for antibiotic resistance. A classic example is the vector pBR322, as shown in Figure 11.5.

The pBR322 plasmid has a size of 4363 base pairs, which enables it to be purified relatively easily. It is used to transform *E. coli* cells which are very commonly used in molecular genetics, and it also exists inside the cells at a relatively high **copy number**, perhaps 20 copies of the plasmid per cell, which also aids its purification.

Figure 11.5 *The plasmid vector pBR322. The positions of the genes encoding antibiotic resistance, the origin of replication and a portion of the site of restriction endonuclease activity are shown*

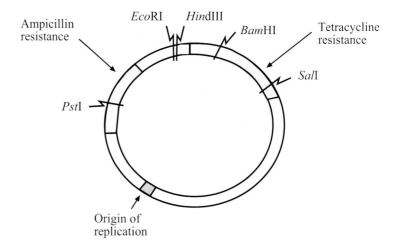

Lastly, it contains two genes which confer on the *E. coli* resistance to the antibiotics ampicillin and tetracycline. Therefore, cells which do or do not have the plasmid are easy to select. Cells are simply transformed with the plasmid and then grown in the presence of one of the antibiotics. Cells which never took up the plasmid lack the resistance genes and therefore will not thrive. Cells which did take up the plasmid will contain the resistance genes and therefore will survive. However, when the inserted DNA is ligated into the plasmid in the first steps of cloning, it is a random event and there is a high chance that the plasmid will be re-ligate back together again with no insert present. The fact that the transformed cells simply have antibiotic resistance does not tell the researcher whether the plasmids are simply wild-type plasmids or those with the desired insert inside. To get over this problem other markers have also been developed.

A common marker for selecting cells which not only have the plasmid inside but also a plasmid containing the DNA of interest has been developed using the *lacZ'* gene. This gene encodes for the enzyme β-galactosidase, but also at one end of the gene is a cluster of restriction enzyme cut sites which can be used for insertion of the insert DNA. Cells are then grown in the presence of an antibiotic, as well as **IPTG** (isopropyl-thiogalactoside) which induces the expression of the *lac* genes, as discussed in Chapter 7, and X-Gal (5-bromo-4-chloro-3-indolyl-β-D-galactopyranoside). This last compound is a substrate for the β-galactosidase produced from the *lac* genes. β-galactosidase turns the X-Gal blue. Therefore, using this type of vector, of which pUC8 is an example, one can end up with various results:

- Cells which do not contain plasmids and are therefore killed by the antibiotic.
- Cells which contain the plasmid but no insert. β-galactosidase will be produced because of the IPTG and the X-Gal will be

turned blue. Therefore the bacterial colonies will appear blue. These colonies are not wanted and will be ignored.

- Cells which contain the plasmid and have the insert in. The DNA will be inserted into the *lac* gene and therefore no β-galactosidase will be made, no blue colour produced and the bacterial colonies will appear white. These are the bacteria that are desired and are identifiable simply by the colour.

There are, of course, presently many different plasmid vectors. Some of these plasmid vectors will be used for the expression of the gene of interest and therefore the desired promoters will also need to be present. However, plasmids can also be limited in their use. The maximum size of the inserted DNA is commonly approximately 8 kb. Therefore, for larger DNA fragments other vectors may be required.

Bacteriophages as vectors

Bacteriophages may also be used as vectors. One of the steps involved in cloning is the reintroduction of the vector back into the host cells. This is often difficult, but here, with bacteriophages, we have a system in which the machinery is already present to do this step for us. Bacteriophages by nature introduce foreign DNA into bacterial cells.

Bacteriophages can also commonly accommodate larger DNA fragments than plasmids, perhaps up to 25 kb. The λ phage has a genome of 49.5 kb, and large parts of this can be removed without the normal functioning of the phage being affected. However, the head size of the phage only allows DNA of less than approximately 52 kb to fit. Therefore, by leaving enough of the phage genome intact for normal functions, there is enough room for an insert of up to about 25 kb.

Like plasmids many variations of the λ phage have been used as vectors. Some variations prevent the phage entering the lysogenic pathway and therefore force it to be lytic. Other variations include selectable markers as we discussed with the plasmids.

A second phage which is commonly used as a vector is the M13. This is a filamentous virus which has a circular genome of 6.4 kb. However, M13 is interesting for two reasons. Firstly, the genome is single-stranded and secondly, the virus particles are released from the host cells without the host cells being killed. Therefore large amounts of the M13 can be grown and harvested, yielding large quantities of the insert DNA in a single-stranded form. Such DNA is useful for sequencing reactions.

Cosmids

Cosmids are a cross between phage vectors and plasmids. These vectors contain the phage cos sites (cohesive ends), which form overhangs at the end of the genome when it is in the linear form, and also contain DNA from plasmids, including the origin of replication and, commonly, genes for antibiotic resistance. These constructs will be packaged into phage particles, for example into the λ phage, in an *in vitro* packaging system, where the coat proteins are supplied from elsewhere. Therefore, the vector DNA is kept extremely small, allowing more insert DNA to be packaged into the phage head. Hence the insert may be as large as 44 kb.

Gene libraries

The strategies for cloning a gene outlined and discussed above assume that a single gene is of interest, and that the relevant DNA has been isolated and then cloned. However, the same technology can be used in the search for new genes. Here, the aim is to clone representative examples of all the DNA in the system of interest, and to then have a way of selectively accessing this. Such systems are known as **gene libraries**.

One of the common types of gene library is the **genomic library**. Here, representative examples of all the DNA in a genome are found in a collection of vectors, which can be separated and screened. A typical strategy for making and using a library is shown in Figure 11.6.

An alternative library can be made using RNA, or more specific-

Complete genome

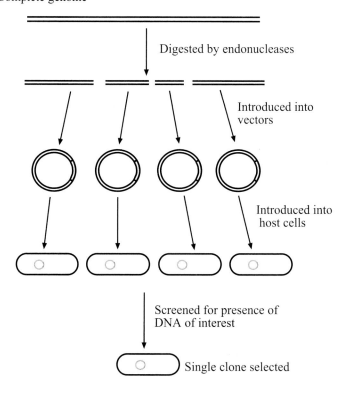

Figure 11.6 *Outline of the strategy for preparing a genomic library*

ally mRNA, as a starting material. This library will not end up containing bits of all the genome, but rather only the genes which are being expressed at the time that the cells are isolated for making the library. Such a library is known as a **cDNA (complementary DNA) library**. The strategy for making such a library is shown in Figure 11.7.

Purified RNA cannot itself be used to make the library, so the first task is to make a DNA copy of the RNA – so-called **complementary DNA or cDNA**. This can be carried out using **reverse transcriptase**, one of the enzymes encoded by and used by retroviruses. The DNA is then made double-stranded and can be ligated into an appropriate vector.

One of the crucial aspects of such a strategy is the quality of the

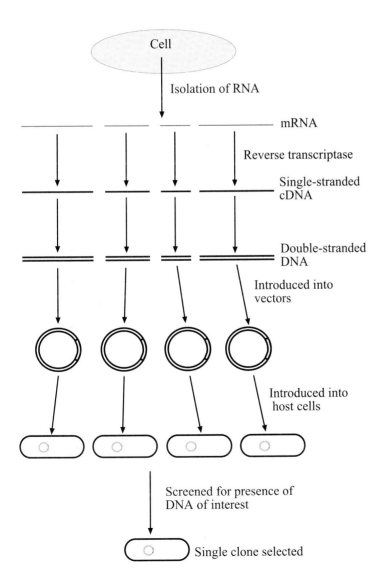

Figure 11.7 *Outline of the strategy for preparing a cDNA library, starting with mRNA*

original mRNA. This must not be degraded. Ideally, the RNA should be intact and therefore the cDNA will be a copy of the whole length of the gene. When the library is screened it is hoped that the gene selected will be of full length. Otherwise other methods would be needed to hunt down the ends of the genes that are missing.

Secondly, as the library is prepared using mRNA from cells which are expressing only a selected number of genes at that moment in time, it may be possible to induce certain cells to preferentially express the gene of interest. Therefore, this might maximize the chances of finding the gene of interest. Clearly, the reverse of this is that the cells might not be expressing the gene of interest at all, and therefore a cDNA library will be of no use.

Probing of libraries

Once a library has been created, the next challenge is to select, out of the vast array of clones, the correct one. This is analogous to going to a real library and selecting out only one book on a particular subject of interest. Clearly, the first thing to do is display all the books in a way in which they can be seen; in a real library they are put on shelves, and not left in boxes. With genetic libraries, the vectors are used to transform cells, and each cell will hopefully contain multiple copies of only one vector, containing its own unique inserted DNA. Therefore, taking *E. coli* as an example, the cells may be plated out on agar and grown. Each resulting colony will stem from one single cell and therefore be identical, each containing the same inserted DNA. Therefore, we have spread out the library and now need to select which colony has the correct piece of DNA. A common strategy is to then make a copy of the *E. coli* colonies which can be used for the selection procedure, leaving the original colonies as a method of keeping the correct cells for later use. For this purpose, a filter of nitrocellulose or a similar material is carefully put over the colonies on the agar, adding marks to enable the nitrocellulose to be realigned later. A proportion of the cells will attach to the nitrocellulose, while the remainder will stay on the agar. A copy of the colonies has been made.

The nitrocellulose is then treated, including a step using either UV light or 80°C for 2 hours, to fix the DNA onto the nitrocellulose and make sure that it is not lost during subsequent treatments.

The nitrocellulose filter is then probed. Probes can be of various types, but commonly a probe is prepared from another fragment of DNA which has the base sequence of interest. Therefore, the base sequence of the probe will then hybridize with a sequence from one fragment, or possibly more, of the inserted DNA in the vectors of the library. The probes are commonly labelled with radioactivity, usually ^{32}P. Thus, on the nitrocellulose will be the vector DNA with inserts, and some of these will have hybridized to the radioactive probe. **Autoradiography**, as discussed in Chapter 10, can now be

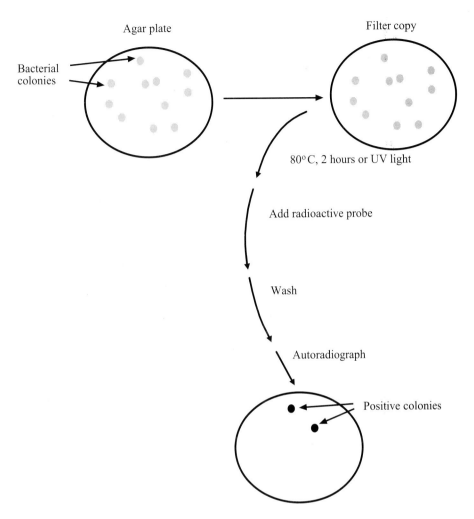

Figure 11.8   *Steps taken in probing a DNA library. The final filter would then be realigned with the original agar plate to identify the colonies of interest*

used to identify which vectors, and therefore which colonies, contain the hybridized probe. Once these colonies have been identified, because the nitrocellulose was a copy of the original agar plate, the colonies on the agar can be identified, grown and used for further DNA purification. A scheme for probing is shown in Figure 11.8.

Often when one is trying to search for a gene, either from the cDNA library or from a genomic library, there is no knowledge of any part of the gene sequence, and therefore designing nucleotide probes is problematical if not impossible. Often in this situation, the protein has been totally or partially purified, and perhaps some amino acid sequence is therefore known. However, it is not a simple case of deducing the nucleotide sequence because, as discussed in Chapter 6, several amino acids have more than one codon. Serine

A nucleotide probe may be a cloned gene, perhaps removed from its vector by restriction enzymes. Alternatively, probes may have been produced by PCR (see Chapter 12) or synthesized as a short oligonucleotide. The longer the probe, however, the better it is likely to work and the more specific the result.

Figure 11.9 *Sequences of three degenerate probes. These differ at positions 3, 5 and 13*

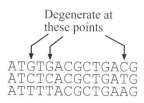

Degenerate at these points

```
ATGTGACGCTGACG
ATCTCACGCTGATG
ATTTTACGCTGAAG
```

> Antibodies to be used for probing may be raised against purified proteins, or raised against a small peptide synthesized using the known amino acid sequence of the protein.

for example has six codons. Therefore deducing the nucleotide sequence from the amino acid sequence, a process referred to as **back-translation,** leaves one with a problem: that of which codon to pick? Several species have a preferred codon usage, and tables of such preferences are available on databases. However, probes need to be made which have all options, and such probes are called **degenerate probes.** Examples are given in Figure 11.9. Typically, areas of the protein can be chosen where the options are minimized; for example, methionine has only one codon and thus there will be no degeneracy here.

The last scenario that we shall discuss here is one in which no sequence information for the gene or the gene product is known. Even here probing is still possible. If an antibody has been raised against the protein, either a polyconal or monoclonal antibody, then this may be used for library probing. However, the vectors into which the DNA fragments have been inserted will have to be different here. Antibodies will only recognize the protein products produced from the gene sequence and, thus, for there to be anything for the antibody to recognize, the proteins will have to be expressed. The DNA fragments or cDNA will need to be inserted into a suitable expression vector, where the host cells recognize the promoter sequences and express the proteins.

Suggested further reading

Brown, T.A. (1995). *Gene Cloning: An Introduction*, 3rd edn. Chapman and Hall. (An excellent text, well worth reading.)

Collins, J. and Hohn, B. (1978). Cosmids: a type of plasmid gene cloning vector that is packagable *in vitro* in bacteriophage heads. *Proceedings of the National Academiy of Sciences, USA,* **75,** 4242–4246.

Glover, D.M., ed. (1985). *DNA Cloning: A Practical Approach.* IRL.

Lathe, R. (1985). Synthetic oligonucleotide probes deduced from amino acid sequence data. Theoretical and practical considerations. *Journal of Molecular Biology,* **183,** 1–12.

Maniatis, T., Hardison, R.C., Lacy, E., Lauer, J., O'Connell, C., Quon, D., Sim, G.K. and Efstratiadis, A. (1978). The isolation of structural genes from libraries of eukaryotic DNA. *Cell,* **15,** 687–701.

Sambrook, J., Fritsch, E.F. and Maniatis, T. (1989). *Molecular*

Cloning: A Laboratory Manual, 2nd edn. Cold Spring Harbor Laboratory Press.

Smith, D.H. (1979). Nucleotide sequence specificity of restriction enzymes. *Science,* 205, 455.

Watson, J.D., Gilman, M., Witkowski, J. and Zoller, M. (1992). *Recombinant DNA,* 2nd edn. Scientific American Books.

Self-assessment questions

1. Name two methods that can be used for DNA isolation.
2. Who invented ultracentrifugation and whose name is now used as a unit to quantify the method?
3. Name two types of ultracentrifugation that can be used for DNA isolation.
4. Which enzymes are used to cut DNA?
5. Which enzymes are used to rejoin DNA?
6. You have used a vector with the *lacZ'* gene and have grown your cells in the presence of IPTG and X-Gal. You now have blue colonies and white colonies. Which colour of colony are you interested in and why?
7. Name one advantage of using a bacteriophage over a plasmid as a vector.
8. Briefly, what is a cosmid?
9. What is a cDNA library?
10. What is the process of deriving a DNA sequence from an amino acid sequence called?
11. From which organism was *Eco*RI isolated and how do we know that from its name?

Key Concepts and Facts

Cloning
- Cloning involves several steps, the use of a vector and the use of a host cell.
- Cloning techniques require the cutting and rejoining of DNA.

DNA Manipulation
- DNA can be isolated by several methods including phenol extraction and centrifugation.
- Ultracentrifugation of DNA may be density gradient centrifugation or velocity centrifugation.
- DNA may be cut at specific points by restriction endonucleases.
- Restriction endonucleases may cut in such a way as to form blunt ends or sticky ends, depending on the enzyme.
- The naming of restriction endonucleases is systematic, and includes elements indicating the organism used for isolation and its strain.
- DNA can be characterized by restriction maps.
- DNA can be joined by ligases – a process known as ligation.

Cloning Vectors
- Vectors need to have sites for the insertion of the DNA of interest, and be selectable.
- Plasmids are commonly used as cloning vectors.
- Often plasmids contain genes which confer antibiotic resistance and this is used for selection.
- A common selection mechanism is the inclusion of the β-galactosidase gene, which can be interrupted by inclusion of the inserted DNA.
- Bacteriophages are often used as vectors and have the advantage of an intrinsic mechanism for DNA entry into the bacteria.
- Cosmids are a cross between plasmids and bacteriophages.

Gene Libraries
- Gene libraries can be used to select a particular DNA sequence.
- Gene libraries may be constructed from genomic DNA or cDNA.
- Gene libraries are commonly probed by the use of a short DNA fragment or oligonucleotide.
- If no DNA sequence data is known, libraries may still be probed by oligonucleotides or antibodies.

Chapter 12
Polymerase chain reaction (PCR)

Learning objectives

After studying this chapter you should confidently be able to:

Describe the technique of polymerase chain reaction (PCR).

Outline some of the considerations needed when designing primers for the polymerase chain reaction.

Appreciate some of the uses of the polymerase chain reaction.

One of the major advances in molecular genetics has been the development of a technique which allows the rapid and relatively cheap amplification of the amount of DNA present in a sample. This technique is called **polymerase chain reaction**, or PCR. The methodology was first devised by Kary Mullis in 1984, but has become widely and extensively used in virtually every molecular genetics laboratory.

The technique of PCR

The essence of the technique is the amplification of a selected area of the DNA sequence of interest. As the unique element of any segment of DNA is its sequence, then areas of this sequence can be targetted and complementary sequences can be designed. This is illustrated in Figure 12.1.

Once the areas of sequence are chosen the complementary sequences can be made chemically, yielding small oligonucleotides

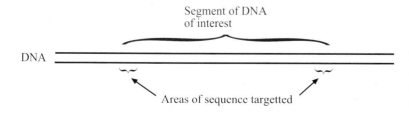

Figure 12.1 *Polymerase chain reaction amplifies only specific regions of DNA, dictated by the design of the primers either side of the area of interest*

called **primers**. These are used to start the new DNA synthesis, as will be seen later.

The reactions can now be carried out to produce the new DNA. The essential elements needed are:

- A pair of primers as described either side of the DNA sequence of interest.
- All four deoxyribonucleoside triphosphates (dNTPs).
- A polymerase to carry out the reaction.

However, it is not simply a case of adding these to a tube and heating. The process takes place in a cyclic manner, where the cycle has three steps:

- Step 1: Heating to 95°C. A denaturing step. This separates the DNA strands and therefore allows the primers to later hybridize to their respective parts of the DNA.
- Step 2: The mixture is rapidly cooled to approximately 54°C. This allows the primers to hybridize to the relevant DNA stretches. The temperature is dictated by the primers, particularly their length and their content of the bases G and C. Variations here include the gradual alteration of this temperature in successive cycles, which can alter the specificity of the hybridization reaction and maximize the chances of obtaining the correct product.
- Step 3: Reheating to 72°C. This is the optimal temperature for DNA synthesis, and it is during this step that the new DNA is made. The length of time at this temperature may be altered depending on the length of the DNA being produced.

The process is depicted in Figure 12.2. In this figure the DNA has been denatured and a single strand is shown for simplicity. The first primer will anneal at the appropriate point in the cycle and then this primer will act as a starting point for the polymerase and a new complementary strand will be produced. In the second cycle this new DNA is separated into separate strands by the high temperature part of the cycle, which allows the annealing of both primers at their appropriate points on the DNA during the next cooling cycle. The polymerase can then produce new complementary strands to both the DNA strands, doubling the amount of DNA. The third cycle will once again denature the DNA, primers will anneal, and the polymerase will once again double the amount of DNA present. This can continue, and typically a reaction may have between 25 and 35 cycles. Therefore, the total amount of DNA produced will be, theoretically, 2^{35} copies of the original DNA in 35 cycles. That is, if we start with 1 molecule of DNA, after 35 cycles we will have nearly 3.5×10^{10} molecules with the same DNA sequence present. In theory, PCR can be achieved with one cell as the starting material, but in practice, the researcher usually starts with much more than that. In addition, the PCR product obtained can be purified and a

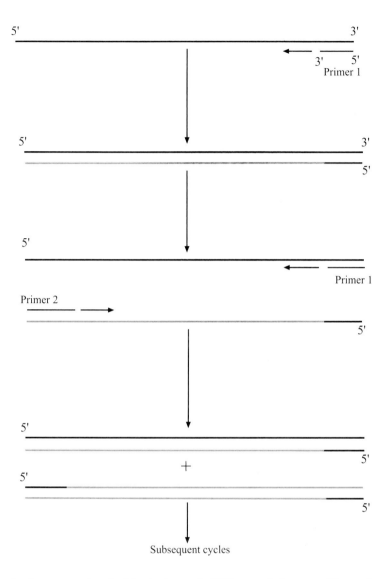

5'
3'
3' 5'
Primer 1

5'
3'
5'

5'

Primer 1

Primer 2

5'

5'

5'

+

5'

5'

Subsequent cycles

Figure 12.2 *Cycles in a polymerase chain reaction. Here we start with single-stranded DNA for clarity, but the same applies to double-stranded DNA too*

further round of 35 cycles of PCR carried out. Thus the amplification is huge. A warning here is that the more cycles and rounds of PCR that are carried out, the greater the number of errors that will be introduced. The polymerase can make mistakes and if this happens and then further rounds of PCR are carried out, the errors are also amplified.

In the early years of PCR, the process was achieved by transferring the tubes of the sample from different water baths set at the required temperatures, but modern machinery with built-in heaters and refrigerators and complicated software has now taken over, and commonly the researcher can set up a PCR experiment and go home for the night, in the sound knowledge that, short of a power cut, the process will be complete in the morning. Such machines are known a **thermal cyclers**, commonly referred to as PCR machines.

Thermal cyclers are now common in nearly all modern biology laboratories. They vary in design and specifications, but essentially they all carry out the same process. More expensive models allow, for example, the times taken between temperatures to be varied, and can have quite complicated temperature cycles. Such variations allow PCR to be even more powerful and to be used in situations where, perhaps a few years ago, results would have been unobtainable.

Figure 12.3 *Real results from a PCR experiment. (Kindly supplied by Dr Radhika Desikan, UWE)*

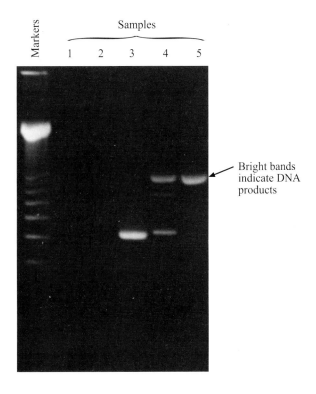

Bright bands indicate DNA products

The final result of the polymerase chain reaction can be analysed by **gel electrophoresis,** as described in Chapter 10. This is usually agarose-based electrophoresis. An example of such an experiment is shown in Figure 12.3. Here it can be seen that certain controls are also included (lanes 1 and 2), for example where the reaction is carried out in the absence of added DNA to ensure that no contamination has taken place. It is easy to amplify an erroneous DNA molecule, the amplification achieved being so great.

However, it must be remembered that it is only the DNA which lies between the DNA primers that will be amplified; any other part of the sequence will, in theory, be ignored. This really highlights the power of the technique. Out of a large amount of DNA, perhaps a whole genome, a small and selected sequence of the DNA can be specifically targetted and amplified. Some more specific examples of this will be discussed below.

As can be seen from the above steps, the mixture is repeatedly heated to near boiling point, and yet, during a subsequent step, we are expecting the enzymatic synthesis of new DNA. How can this be achieved? The secret is that the polymerase that is used in this reaction is isolated from an organism which lives happily at very high temperatures and therefore its enzymes are heat resistant for some reason. Archaebacteria, for example, from the Yellowstone National Park, are able to live at temperatures above 90°C. Organisms which are able to survive such high temperatures are known as **thermophiles** and much interest has been generated in trying to understand what it is about the protein structure of these organisms that allows them to function at these temperatures. Normally a protein would become denatured at less than 60°C.

The enzyme of interest here is polymerase from *Thermus aquaticus*, and the enzyme is referred to as *Taq* polymerase. It is relatively expensive, but very little is needed in each reaction. Also, new variants which have been genetically engineered are now on the market, making the process better.

How do you target the DNA sequence of interest? To do this, the sequence of interest has to be known, or at least the ends of the sequence need to be known. The primers are then designed with the complementary sequence. But what are the rules governing the design of PCR primers? Here are a few considerations:

- The primers are usually only between 18 and 20 base pairs long and are therefore relatively cheap to produce.
- The primers need to be a certain distance apart, usually between 200 bases and 600 bases. This is governed by the length of new DNA that the polymerase can produce without problems occurring, although more recently longer sequences can be amplified with modified polymerases.
- The primers need to be designed against both the strands of the DNA.
- The primers need to be designed so that they face each other.
- The primers need to be unique. Ideally, the sequence the primers have been designed around should not occur elsewhere in the DNA that is used as the starting material, otherwise the wrong part of the DNA may be amplified.
- The primers must not anneal to each other.
- The C/G content of the primers is important and may help decide the annealing temperatures used during the cycles.

Some of these rules are illustrated in Figure 12.4.

If the secret as to why proteins from thermophiles can resist such high temperatures can be found, then the structures can be genetically engineered into new proteins of interest to industry. Presently, if an enzyme is used in an industrial process, relatively low temperatures are needed to prevent the enzyme being denatured. However, if the protein could be used at higher temperatures, then reaction rates would be increased and so would the rate of product generation – obviously of interest to the industries involved.

In theory, a PCR product can be obtained if only one molecule of original DNA exists. However, such power has its drawbacks. Because amplification is so great, it is too easy to amplify contaminating DNA, and this has to be controlled for.

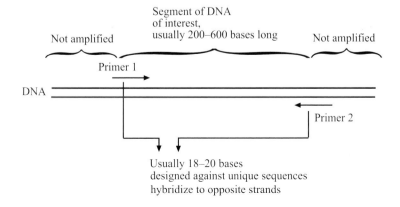

Figure 12.4 *Designing PCR primers. Some of the considerations that need to be borne in mind before ordering or making specific primer sequences*

Some of the uses of polymerase chain reaction

The above discussion explains how PCR works and highlights the power it gives the molecular geneticist. But what are the sorts of things the technique is used for?

Finding genes in genomes

One of the powerful uses of PCR is to look for the presence of a gene or DNA sequence within a genome. It may be that one researcher has found the presence of a gene in one species, but would like to know if it is also present in other species. Or perhaps one enzyme has been found and it is thought that many forms of the enzyme exist. By designing the primers correctly, other forms of the enzyme may be revealed. Therefore, once the sequence is known, PCR can be used to 'fish out' the sequence from another source. However, it must be remembered that your resulting product will only be formed between the two designed PCR primers, and therefore the result may be well short of a full-length gene product. To find the full length, perhaps the researcher will then screen a library with the PCR product as described in Chapter 11.

Finding a gene within the genome may also be useful in the technique of **transgenics**, as discussed more fully in Chapter 14. Here, a gene is placed in a genome artificially, but the techniques are far from certain, and there is a high chance that the gene will not be integrated into the genome, or will be integrated incorrectly. Again with the use of PCR, the new gene, known as the **transgene**, may be confirmed to be present or absent in the genome of the transgenic animal and, again with the correct design of primers, the PCR may be used to verify the integration into the correct part of the genome.

Comparisons of genomes

It is useful sometimes to be able to compare genomes, and perhaps discover how closely related two species might be. Such information may be obtained by a technique known as **random amplified polymorphic DNA (RAPD) analysis**. Here, random PCR primers are used, with the result that many DNA products are formed and the resulting gel will have many bands. It is then a case of analysing the banding pattern obtained to look for similarities. A very oversimplified version is given in Figure 12.5.

Clinical uses

PCR may be used very advantageously in a clinical setting too. Suspected mutations within genes or more gross genome alterations may be found by amplification of certain regions of genes and then

Species 1   Species 2   Species 3

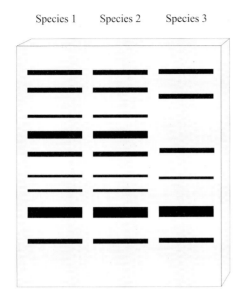

Figure 12.5 *Simplified example of the results from a random amplified polymorphic DNA analysis (RAPD analysis). Species 1 and 2 show the same pattern and are therefore related. Species 3 shows a different banding pattern and is therefore much less related*

sequencing or analysis on gels. Alternatively, the presence of viruses, such as HIV (human immunodeficiency virus) which causes AIDS (acquired immune deficiency syndrome), may be determined in small samples of blood by, in this case, designing PCR primers to the HIV sequence.

Degenerate PCR

In the above discussion the sequence of the gene or segment of DNA was known, and therefore designing of the relevant DNA primers was relatively simple. However, this is not always the case. It may be that the only sequence known for a particular enzyme is the amino acid sequence. Returning down the pathway of protein synthesis and trying to determine the nucleotide sequence from the amino acid sequence is not always very easy, especially when it is remembered that some amino acids have many codons. Therefore the primers may have to have variations within them and such primers are known as **degenerate primers**. This problem was also discussed in Chapter 11 and examples of degenerate DNA sequences are shown in Figure 11.9. Clearly, the conditions of the cycles in the PCR will need to be altered to take into account the degenerate nature of the primers, and the technique does not always yield sensible results.

Degenerate PCR may also be used for finding other forms of the same gene. If it is suspected that many forms of the same enzyme exist, but little is known about the other forms (perhaps they are in a relatively unrelated species), then degenerate primers may help in the search.

If PCR is used in a clinical environment, to look for an inherited genetic defect or the presence of a virus, for example, then this information can be used to advise individuals on subsequent actions, such as AIDS patients and their relationships or whether a couple should try for a baby.

RT-PCR

In Chapter 10 we discussed the way in which a researcher may determine if a gene is expressed, perhaps under certain conditions or in certain tissues of the organism. Northern blotting, as discussed, is a very powerful technique for this purpose but it has one major drawback, and that is sensitivity. An alternate method is to use **reverse transcriptase-polymerase chain reaction**, so-called RT-PCR.

In RT-PCR we are looking for the presence of RNA in a sample, but using DNA amplification to achieve this. How can this be done? Firstly, the RNA has to be copied into a DNA molecule. This can be done by the use of the enzyme reverse transcriptase. This enzyme is used by retroviruses (RNA viruses) in their normal life cycle. They need to turn the RNA into a DNA copy before it can be integrated into the genome of the host. Here we can use the same rationale to turn the RNA isolated from cells into a DNA copy. However, the RNA may be very scarce within the sample, perhaps only one or a few copies in total. We can then design and use PCR primers against the RNA sequence of interest to determine if the RNA was originally present. A scheme to illustrate this is given in Figure 12.6. The results are once again revealed by gel electrophoresis. An example of a research project using this technique is given in the suggested further reading.

Quantification of PCR

One of the major problems of PCR is that of quantification. With Northern blotting, as described in Chapter 10, densitometry can be used to scan the resulting photographs, but with PCR it is hard to achieve a measure of the quantity. The production of the new DNA is basically exponential, but will then start to tail off as the number of cycles is pushed too high. Very few laboratories have cycle numbers beyond 40, as by this time erroneous synthesis takes place and the process starts to falter. Therefore it is very hard to know exactly what amplification has taken place and therefore virtually impossible to know the amount of starting DNA with the correct sequence. In RT-PCR, a researcher often reports a total lack in certain samples and a presence in other samples, with very little attempt at quantification. However, methods are being published that include quantification, and putting numbers to the concentration of DNA using PCR will undoubtedly become more common in the future.

Because of the power of amplification afforded by PCR, it is a technique that is being used to hunt for DNA from dinosaurs, in a *Jurassic Park* type scenario. Insects which have been feeding off dinosaur blood have been found in embedded amber from trees. Subsequently, the DNA can be extracted from the insect and amplified using PCR. However, contamination problems have thrown great doubt over such work, and few people believe that DNA can in fact survive the several millions of years required to actually be from dinosaurs.

Suggested further reading

Arnheim, N. and Erlich, H. (1992). Polymerase chain reaction strategy. *Annual Review of Biochemistry*, **61**, 131–156.

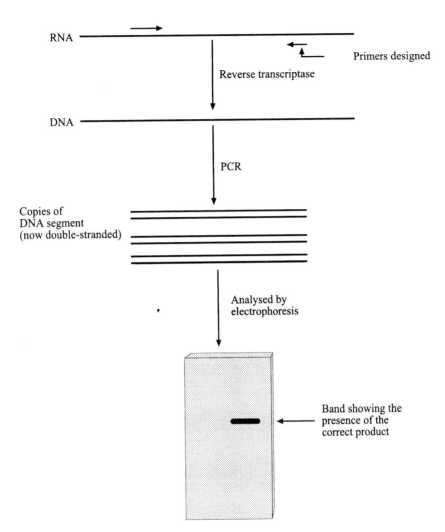

Figure 12.6 *Scheme showing the steps needed in reverse transcriptase-PCR (RT-PCR)*

RT-PCR

In Chapter 10 we discussed the way in which a researcher may determine if a gene is expressed, perhaps under certain conditions or in certain tissues of the organism. Northern blotting, as discussed, is a very powerful technique for this purpose but it has one major drawback, and that is sensitivity. An alternate method is to use **reverse transcriptase-polymerase chain reaction**, so-called RT-PCR.

In RT-PCR we are looking for the presence of RNA in a sample, but using DNA amplification to achieve this. How can this be done? Firstly, the RNA has to be copied into a DNA molecule. This can be done by the use of the enzyme reverse transcriptase. This enzyme is used by retroviruses (RNA viruses) in their normal life cycle. They

Mullis, K.B., Ferré, F. and Gibbs, R.A., eds. (1994). *The Polymerase Chain Reaction.* Birkhaüser.

Ryuchlik, W., Spencer, W.J. and Rhoads, R.E. (1990). Optimization of the annealing temperature for DNA amplification *in vitro. Nucleic Acids Research*, **18**, 6409–6412.

Saiki, R.K., Gelfand, D.H., Stoffel, S., Scharf, S., Higuchi, R., Horn, G.T., Millis, K.B. and Erlich, H.A. (1988). Primer-directed enzymatic amplification of DNA with a thermostable DNA polymerase. *Science*, **239**, 487–491.

Self-assessment questions

1. How is the specificity of the amplification of PCR achieved?
2. List the three main steps needed to achieve the polymerase chain reaction.
3. Once the PCR has been completed, how is the resulting DNA analysed?
4. Which enzyme is usually used for the synthesis of the DNA in PCR?
5. When designing primers for PCR, there are several considerations that need to be taken into account. One of these is the length of the final product, i.e. the distance between the primers. What does this distance usually range between?
6. Why is PCR useful for a researcher carrying out transgenics?
7. What does the abbreviation RT-PCR stand for?
8. What is RT-PCR used for?
9. If 20 cycles of PCR are carried out on one molecule of original DNA, how many molecules of DNA will be present at the end?
10. Name one use of random amplified polymorphic DNA analysis (RAPD analysis).

Key Concepts and Facts

Polymerase Chain Reaction

- Polymerase chain reaction (PCR) is an extremely powerful technique for the amplification of the amount of DNA present.

- The key elements for PCR are a pair of oligonucleotide primers, dNTPs and a polymerase.

- The three steps of PCR are denaturation, reannealing of primers and synthesis.

- PCR doubles the DNA present for each cycle.

- The polymerase usually used is from a thermophilic organism, *Thermus aquaticus*.

- Primers need to be carefully designed to ensure maximum specificity and maximum success.

- Contamination can easily be amplified too!

Uses of PCR

- PCR can be used to find genes in genomes.

- Comparisons of genomes can be carried out with PCR.

- PCR can be used to find defects in genes which cause disease.

- The presence of viruses or bacteria in a patient can be found by PCR.

- PCR can be made less specific by the use of degenerative primers.

- Gene expression and RNA can be determined by RT-PCR.

- Methods have been devised to quantify PCR, although at present they are not commonly used.

Chapter 13
Sequencing and sequence analysis

Learning objectives

After studying this chapter you should confidently be able to:

Explain why obtaining DNA sequence information is important.

Describe the methods of obtaining DNA sequences.

Outline the information that may be obtained about a new sequence.

Explain how we might ascertain whether a sequence obtained contains the complete open reading frame.

Explain how one might determine the correct reading frame of an unknown sequence.

Describe how one might determine if the same DNA sequence or a similar one has been reported by another researcher.

Describe the information that accompanies a sequence logged in the international databases.

Explain how to gain insight into the possible structure of a protein encoded by a gene.

Explore the Internet to discover the facilities available to today's molecular geneticist.

One of the major challenges in molecular genetics lies in understanding how the whole genome functions to create and maintain the survival of the organism. To do this, it would be of great advantage if the sequence of the whole genome of an organism was known, and therefore all the genes within that genome identified. Once this is done, it should be possible to identify all the proteins expressed by that genome, and therefore all the machinery of the organism will have been identified, even if we still don't know how much of it works. To this end, several genomes have been completely sequenced, while large projects are underway to sequence others. Genomes which have been completely sequenced include those of *Haemophilus influenzae*, *Saccharomyces cerevisiae*, *Helicobacter pylori*, *Escherichia coli* and *Bacillus subtilis*. Others which are being sought include those of the fruit fly (*Drosophila melanogaster*), the model plant *Arabidopsis thaliana*, rice (*Oryza sativa*), the mouse (*Mus musculis*), the rat (*Rattus norvegicus*) and humans (the **Human Genome Project**). This last project involves the collaboration of laboratories in Japan, the USA and Europe with the aim of completing the sequencing of the human genome by 2005. However, it should be borne in mind that the sequence obtained from the project will represent that carried by certain members of the population, and will not be identical for everyone. We all carry polymorphisms and mutations in redundant regions of our DNA, but the crucial and functioning parts of our genomes should at least be very similar.

Sequencing

Over the years many methods and modifications have been developed to identify the sequence of a length of DNA. One of these methods was developed by Allan Maxam and Walter Gilbert (the **Maxam–Gilbert method**). Here, the DNA is radiolabelled at one end and is then specifically cleaved in separate reactions at one of the four nucleotides, that is, at C, G, A or T. The fragments so created are then separated by gel electrophoresis and the sequence revealed by the size of the fragments created by each reaction.

However, the most common method used was developed by Frederick Sanger and his associates, the so-called **Sanger dideoxy method**. Here, single-stranded DNA is used as a template and polymerase used to synthesize a copy. This process requires a short oligonucleotide primer and this can be made chemically, a step commonly achieved by the use of a machine called an **oligonucleotide synthesizer**. With very large lengths of DNA the start site of sequencing can be chosen by designing the primer to hybridize to the correct part of the DNA. The polymerase reaction is carried out in the presence of radiolabelled nucleotides to allow the results to be revealed by autoradiography. Also in the reaction mixture is an analogue of one of the nucleotides. This is a $2'$-$3'$ dideoxy analogue which lacks the $3'$-hydroxyl group needed in the formation of the next phosphodiester bond during synthesis (see Figure 13.1). Therefore, when the polymerase incorporates this analogue into the growing chain, no further chain extension can take place. This event will be random and, thus, if it is the adenine analogue that is used, chain termination will take place at any point along the chain at which an A should be incorporated. Hence, by setting up four such reactions, one for each of the four nucleotides, all the possible chain terminations will take place. Therefore the four reactions have created all possible copies of the original DNA,

Walter Gilbert was born in 1932 and obtained a PhD in mathematics from Cambridge, USA, in 1957. In 1980 he was awarded the Nobel prize for Chemistry for his contribution to molecular biology.

Figure 13.1 *Chemical structure of a 2′-3′ dideoxy analogue of a nucleotide, showing where the hydroxyl group is missing*

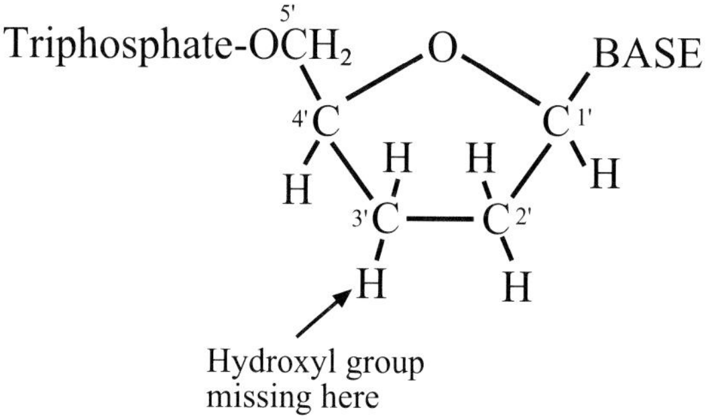

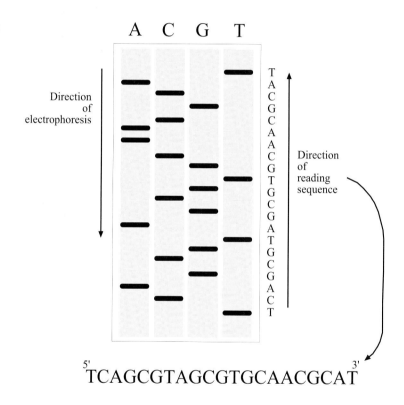

Figure 13.2 *Schematic representation of a sequencing gel, with the sequence underneath*

each terminated at one base further along the chain than the next. All that needs to be done is to analyse the fragments by electrophoresis and the sequence should be able to be read. In practice this involves running a gel, and then autoradiographing it as described in Chapter 10. A schematic of the results is shown in Figure 13.2, while a real gel is shown in Figure 13.3.

Several modifications to this method have been developed. Firstly, the **radiolabel** ^{32}P is routinely used but sharper images are obtained if ^{33}P or ^{35}S is used. Secondly, original sequencing relied on the **Klenow fragment** of polymerase I, but more recently other polymerases are used which allow either longer sequencing runs to be done, or sequencing at higher temperatures, thus avoiding

Frederick Sanger was born in 1918, and studied extensively at Cambridge, UK. He was the first person ever to win the Nobel prize for Chemistry twice: once in 1958 for his work on insulin and again in 1980 for his contribution to DNA sequencing techniques.

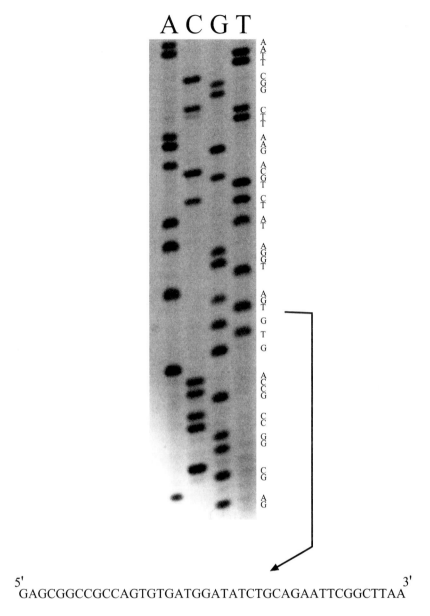

Figure 13.3   *Photograph of a real sequencing gel. (Kindly supplied by Dr Radhika Desikan, UWE)*

possible secondary structures which may interfere with the sequencing. Examples include the phage T7 polymerase, so-called sequenase, or *Taq* polymerase from the thermophilic bacterium *Thermus aquaticus*, as discussed in Chapter 12.

An advance in this technology which has made sequencing much faster is the invention of **automated sequencing equipment**. Here, the same biochemistry is employed, but instead of using radiolabels, the nucleotides are **fluorescently labelled**. By using four different fluorescent labels it is even possible to run all four chain-terminated

DNAs in one lane and still read the sequence. The gel is scanned by a fluorescence detector linked to a computer as the gel is run and thus, as the bands travel past the detector, they are registered. With some sophisticated software the computer can simply report back the sequence to the researcher. The raw data are also captured to enable checks on uncertain parts of the sequence to be made by the researcher. Many laboratories with such equipment will advertise commercial sequencing of other people's DNA, a valuable service to those without automated set-ups.

Sequence analysis

Once the sequence has been obtained, what are the questions that we need to ask which are, perhaps, answerable by modern day sequence analysis?

- Is the sequence complete?
- Is it already known?
- What does it encode?
- Is it homologous to anything else?
- What is the protein's function?
- What does this protein potentially look like?
- Is it modified by the cell?
- Where does it reside in the cell?

Here, an attempt will be made to show that it is possible to obtain significant insight into the answers to these questions. But perhaps it should be noted at this point that many of the answers obtained are predictions and often, therefore, long and complicated experiments are needed to confirm or refute the outcomes of such analysis.

Further manipulation of the DNA sequence

It is often useful to know if or where the fragment of DNA obtained will be cut by restriction enzymes. Computer programs exist, such as the **SEQNET** service at Daresbury, UK, which will find restriction sites for all known restriction enzymes. Such analysis may help in the choosing of the correct enzyme if the DNA fragment is to be inserted into a new cloning vector.

Often DNA fragments obtained are used as probes. Here, the probe needs to be able to hybridize to the DNA of interest, perhaps in a Southern blot, and not to itself. Again, computer programs are available to predict such self-hybridization and the creation of so-called **stem-loop** structures. The same might apply when one is designing PCR primers, because here too stem-loop formation needs to be avoided.

SEQNET and the GCG suite of programs is undergoing a move while this book is in press. In the future, it will be held at the MRC's Human Genome Mapping Project (HGMP) Resource Centre at Hinxton.

Is the sequence complete?

In Part One of this book we discussed the mechanisms of transcription and translation, and these can be used to analyse a sequence obtained. Let us take a length of mRNA as an example. Perhaps we have cloned a DNA fragment which was derived from mRNA isolated from the eukaryotic cell of interest. What does the knowledge about the cell's transcription and translation machinery tell us that we should look for? We know that the majority of eukaryotic mRNA species will have a poly(A) tail at the 3′ end of the molecule. Therefore, when our fragment has been sequenced, can we see evidence of the poly(A) sequence? If we can, then the 3′ end of the original mRNA is represented in our sequence. If not, we are likely to be missing the 3′ end. At the 5′ end we need a start codon from which translation will progress. In eukaryotes, we remember this is always a methionine codon (AUG). In prokaryotes, perhaps we will be looking for a Shine–Dalgarno sequence. If the start codon can be identified then we can start to translate the sequence into a protein sequence. As we move towards the 3′ end we should encounter a stop codon. The region of the sequence between the start codon and the stop codon is the **open reading frame (ORF)** and this gives us the complete sequence of the polypeptide that the gene encodes. Our sequence is therefore complete.

In the above example it was relatively easy to translate the sequence, and because we know the genetic code, such translation can be done by hand by simply reading off the codons. Usually a computer is used, unless the sequence is very short. However, if the start codon is missing, how do we translate the sequence? The answer is that we translate the sequence in every possible way. With a length of double-stranded DNA we therefore have six possible translations and computers can substantially speed up the process. The problem is highlighted by Figure 13.4.

Having obtained our six translations, how do we know which is the right one? The answer is, in fact, often obvious, as there is

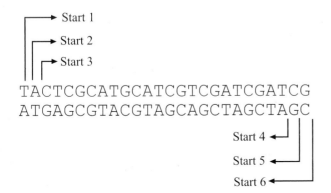

Figure 13.4 *The six possible starts of translation if the start site is not known for a fragment of DNA*

usually only one correct translation. Below are two possible results (out of the six) and it should be obvious that only the second one is correct and has an open reading frame:

T S Z **Met** A **STOP** N V W T K L G Z E Q **STOP** G A R G F P T W R **STOP** A S P R C C **STOP STOP** K M M A R H H I K L I A R N **STOP** E Z G H **STOP**

Met M L I G Z A R D B W T G H E Q R F P L I L E Q A N B D D N H L I P F Z V V Y M M W T B D S P R N R A G G P L I W E G A R T W F P **STOP**

This second sequence starts with a methionine and ends with a stop and, importantly, does not have any other stops in between, giving a reasonably long ORF.

Several translation programs are available on computers either on-line as an interactive session or via the World Wide Web. Most molecular geneticists have use of mainframe computer facilities; for example, in the UK these are at Daresbury. Here the SEQNET service is provided which comprises a host of useful programs, including translation facilities. The results are obtained almost instantaneously and can be saved or transferred to other computers, maybe back to a local PC. Alternatively, Internet sites such as **Expasy** also offer excellent translation facilities. Some of these Internet addresses, but by no means all of them, are listed below.

As well as translation facilities, computers even allow one to go the other way. It is possible with the use of the correct program and a codon usage table to **back-translate** an amino acid sequence into a DNA sequence. Obviously, the DNA sequence will be either degenerate or a best guess, owing to the variability of the codons used to encode some amino acids.

What does it encode?

Once the sequence of the DNA has been obtained, the next question is probably what is it? Commonly the question would be, has anyone else already sequenced it? If they have and a match can be found, the identity of the new sequence will be apparent. Often this question is also asked if probes are being designed for Southern blots, Northern blots or PCR. Here, the probes need to be unique and it is important to check that the sequence chosen is not a common one, lacking the specificity needed.

The main approach to answering these question is to search through all the known data for DNA sequences in the world. This might sound like an impossible task. However, genetics databases located and maintained at several sites around the world hold all the logged genetic sequences known to date. These are continually being expanded, as information from many laboratories is sent in, not least the data from the genome sequencing projects mentioned above. These databases are held in the USA (**Genbank**), in Japan

Many amino acids are encoded by more than one codon, and therefore to back-translate from amino acid sequence to DNA sequence is difficult. However, some species have a preferred use of codons for some amino acids, and by analysis of many sequences from one species, a codon preference table (codon usage table) may be drawn up. This will then be used to optimize the results of an attempted back-translation.

and in Europe (**EMBL**), and each database sources its information from the others on a regular basis so that access to any of these will be equivalent. At the present time, the data held is some 2 330 000 entries!

Segments of the entered sequence of interest to the researcher, perhaps one just sequenced in the laboratory, are scanned across entries in the database, until all parts of the entered sequence have been matched with all parts of the database. Therefore, it can be seen that this is a mammoth task, and clearly would be impossible without a computer. The researcher also has the option to alter certain parameters for searching, such as whether gaps are allowed to find the optimum sequence match.

Therefore, once the individual has completed their sequencing, the databases will allow the researcher to search for known matches. If one is found, or great similarity (homology) is found between the sequence in question and one in the database, the protein or RNA product which is encoded by that gene may be identified.

If a match is found, the information in the entry returned commonly includes, amongst other information:

- **Accession number**: This is a unique code given to the sequence, a bit like the numbers on the spines of books in the library, and therefore can be used for subsequent searching or retrieval of that particular sequence.

- **Title**: Usually tells you what it is, if known, but is usually informative about its origin.

- Papers pertaining to that sequence: If the sequence has been published in established journals, or has been worked on and new information pertaining to that sequence has been published, a list of papers is given. This also, of course, gives you the names of the researcher(s) who originally did the experimentation.

- **Translation**: Commonly a DNA sequence is translated if it encodes a polypeptide.

- Areas of interest within the sequence: If regions of functionality or interest have been identified within the sequence, they are commonly listed.

- The sequence: The DNA sequence is given in full with numbering to help find regions within the sequence.

It may also be wise to translate the sequence and compare this to known protein sequences. Databases for protein sequences also exist; for example, one is called **SWISS-PROT** and presently contains nearly 70 000 sequences. Due to the degenerativeness of the genetic code, the sequences may be relatively different at the DNA level but surprisingly similar at the amino acid level.

However, even if the sequence of interest does not find a match in the database it may still be possible to gain an insight into the likely

A prosthetic group is a non-protein moiety which is part of a protein. A classic example is haem in haemoglobin. Commonly, the part of the protein which interacts with the prosthetic group and holds it in place is very similar in many proteins, some of which might not appear to have much similarity otherwise.

function of the protein simply from the sequence. A database called **Prosite** holds known consensus sequences, currently with 1335 entries, of the most likely sequences found within a protein which will have a certain function. These may be active site regions of enzymes, areas which bind other proteins, or binding sites for prosthetic groups within proteins.

An example of this can be seen when a new protein has been cloned and, for example, is predicted to contain an **EF hand**. This is a protein motif known to bind to Ca^{2+} ions and is found in many proteins that are regulated by intracellular Ca^{2+} levels, for example **calmodulin**. If the new protein contains such an EF hand, the researcher may predict that the protein is also regulated by Ca^{2+} levels, and therefore new experiments may be designed to test this hypothesis. Many proteins have been found to contain receptor motifs when cloned, and these proteins are thought to be receptors. But neither the ligand which activates them nor the downstream signalling pathway has been identified, and therefore such proteins are referred to as **orphan receptors**. Similarly, many proteins have been found to contain kinase active sites, but again their targets for phosphorylation have yet to be identified. It may be, of course, that such predictions are wrong and the predicted motifs are not functional.

What does this protein potentially look like?

Once the sequence of the gene is known and the translated sequence therefore deduced, a prediction of the protein structure can be made. Several computer programs are available to do this, an example being **Peptidestructure**, which is part of the **GCG (Genetic Computer Group)** suite of programs at Daresbury.

This program will return, amongst other information, predictions about:

- Surface probability: Whether regions within the protein are hydrophobic or hydrophilic. This can be very useful in predicting whether a protein is membrane-bound or more likely to be soluble. If it is membrane-bound it may predict how many times it passes through the membrane.
- Antigenicity: Whether regions of the protein are likely to be antigenic and thus can be used to raise antibodies to peptides which may subsequently recognize the full length protein.
- Structure: Certain parameters, such as those worked out by **Chou and Fasman**, amongst others, can be used to predict whether regions of the protein will preferentially fold into α-helices, β-sheets or have turned structures. Of course, such predictions have to be tested experimentally, using perhaps antibody binding, **X-ray diffraction** or **NMR** (nuclear magnetic resonance).

If a protein or other substance is injected into an animal and that animal recognizes it as foreign it will raise antibodies against it. Such substances are said to be antigenic. The computer can predict whether areas of a protein are likely to lead to such a response – the so-called antigenicity index. Small peptides can be synthesized with the amino acid sequences of these antigenic regions and then used to raise antibodies. Usually mice or rabbits are used as the animals for such work.

- Glycosylation: Whether a protein undergoes any post-translational modifications can also be predicted by computer. For example, the consensus sequence recognized by the cell's machinery which adds oligosaccharides to proteins is known and a protein's sequence can be searched for these consensus sequences. However, just because such a potential glycosylation sequence has been found does not mean that it is automatically used by the cell. It may be buried deeply within the protein or within the interior of a membrane and be inaccessible to the enzymes catalysing the modification. Other modifications may also be predicted by sequence analysis.

The last question I wish to address here, but by no means the last addressed by many molecular geneticists, is where in the cell is the protein likely to be. Again the sequence may reveal this information. This is because, when a protein is synthesized, the cell needs to know where it is to be located. The only unique information about the protein synthesized is its sequence and therefore within the sequence an address label is placed. Many of these address labels have now been identified. For example, secretory proteins usually have an N-terminal peptide which is used to direct the protein to the endoplasmic reticulum and beyond. Similarly, proteins destined for location into the mitochondria or chloroplasts have their own unique address within the sequence. The consensus sequences for these addresses can be searched for and may indicate where in the cell the gene's encoded protein may function. Of course, experimentation will once again be needed to confirm such predictions, but this information may be useful in at least confirming or refuting the presence of a gene's encoded protein product in a particular metabolic pathway. If the protein is predicted to be in the wrong place within the cell, perhaps it is not involved after all!

Some useful Internet addresses

The usefulness of the computer has been greatly increased by the introduction of the Internet, and presently several sites are available to those who have access to the Web. Useful sites include BLAST, the international databases, and various sites at many academic institutes which give easy links to useful programs. Here are just a few which the reader may find useful.

Sequence retrieval system (SRSWWW at SEQNET) can be found at:

http://salpha2.dl.ac.uk/srs/srsc

SRSWWW also holds a listing of the databases currently available.

To do a BLAST search:

http://www.ncbi.nlm.nih.gov/cgi-bin/BLAST/nph-blast?Jform=0

The Expasy site:
  http://expasy.hcuge.ch/

To do a Genbank search:
  http://www2.ncbi.nlm.nih.gov./genbank/query_form.html

The Institute for Genomic Research (TIGR):
  http://www.tigr.org/tdb/

Multiple sequence alignments (at ClustalW) can be entered at:
  http://www2.ebi.ac.uk/clustalw/

The Mendel Plant Gene Nomenclature Database homepage:
  http://jiio6.jic.bbsrc.ac.uk/index.html

Other interesting WWW pages concern information from genome projects or particular subjects in genetics. Here are a few of these, but this is far from a definitive list.

Magpie genome sequencing projects:
  http://www.c.mcs.anl.gov/home/genomes/

Human Genome Project information pages:
  http://www.ornl.gov/hgmis/home.html

Genecards – human genes, proteins and diseases:
  http://bioinformatics.weismann.ac.il/cards/

An interesting genetics page can be found at:
  http://www.genetic.org/

The Dog Genome Project:
  http://mendel.berkeley.edu/dog.html

Suggested further reading

Alberts, B., Bray, D., Lewis, J., Raff, M., Roberts, K. and Watson, J.D. (1994). *Molecular Biology of the Cell*, 3rd edn. Garland Press. (Chapter on protein targeting in particular.)

Blattner, F. *et al.* (1997). The complete genome sequence of *Escherichia coli* K-12. *Science*, **277**, 1453–1462.

Branden, G. and Tooze, J. (1999). *Introduction to Protein Structure*, 2nd edn. Garland Press.

Brown, T.A. (1994). *DNA Sequencing*. IRL Press. (A good book for trouble-shooting.)

Fleischmann, R.D. *et al.* (1995). Whole-genome random sequencing and assembly of *Haemophilus influenzae* Rd. *Science*, **269**, 496–512.

Goffeau, A. *et al.* (1996). Life with 6000 genes. *Science*, **274**, 546–567 (*Saccharomyces cerevisiae* genome.)

Jordan, E. and Collins, F.S. (1996). Human Genome Project: a march of genetic maps. *Nature*, **380**, 111–112.

Maxam, A.M. and Gilbert, W. (1977). A new method for sequencing DNA. *Proceedings of the National Academy of Sciences, USA*, **74**, 560–564.

Nucleic Acids Research (1997). **Vol. 25,** No. 1. (A list of specialized databases.)

Sanger, F., Nicklen, S. and Coulson, A.R. (1977). DNA sequencing with chain-terminating inhibitors. *Proceedings of the National Academy of Sciences, USA*, **74**, 5463–5467.

Tomb J.-F. *et al.* (1997). The complete genome sequence of the gastric pathogen *Helicobacter pylori. Nature*, **388**, 539–547.

Self-assessment questions

1. Which method of DNA sequencing uses nucleotide cleavage as its basis?
2. Name the method of sequencing which uses DNA synthesis termination?
3. After a sequencing gel has been run using samples from the Sanger dideoxy method, to read the sequence, which way is the banding pattern read off the gel: from top to bottom or from bottom to top?
4. Automated DNA sequencing does not rely on radioactive labelling. How are the nucleotides commonly labelled in this type of sequencing?
5. What is the open reading frame (ORF) of a gene sequence?
6. If one has a double-stranded DNA fragment with no obvious start site, how many possible ways are there to translate the sequence?
7. Name a protein sequence database.
8. Name a database of consensus sequences.
9. What type of prediction did Chou and Fasman devise?
10. What does the Human Genome Project hope to achieve?

Key Concepts and Facts

Sequencing
- Several genome projects aim to completely sequence genomes from animals such as the mouse, rat and humans.

- Sequencing a DNA fragment obtained or cloned is crucial to identifying it and its use in the cell.

- Sequencing methods include the Maxam–Gilbert method and the Sanger dideoxy method.

- The procedure commonly used today is the Sanger dideoxy method based on synthesis termination.

- Sequencing can be achieved by automated machinery based on fluorescent labelling.

Sequence Analysis
- Various analyses of the sequence will reveal much about the DNA sequence and the protein/product encoded.

- An open reading frame can be identified if present.

- A double-stranded DNA can be translated in six different ways, but only one of these will be the correct way.

- Databases of sequences, such as Genbank, are available on computer via the computer network. These are searchable.

- Prosite is a database of consensus sequences.

- SWISS-PROT is a database of protein sequences.

- Many programs are available for analysis of, amongst other things, restriction endonuclease cut sites, back-translation, or self-hybridization.

- Programs are available on computer to indicate how a protein might fold, or perhaps where it might be located in the cell.

- The Internet is a growing resource for the molecular geneticist, with many sites already on-line.

Chapter 14

The future of molecular genetics: biotechnology, transgenics and gene therapy

Learning objectives

After studying this chapter you should confidently be able to:

Outline the uses to which DNA technology can be put.

Explain the considerations needed to ensure that a gene is expressed in a host organism.

List some products of DNA biotechnology.

Outline the uses of transgenics to agriculture, in both plants and animals.

Describe how transgenic animals are created.

Explain the uses of gene therapy and the obstacles which need to be overcome.

Outline the cloning of animals.

Debate the ethical issues surrounding modern molecular genetics.

Within this book we have discussed the mechanisms by which DNA is replicated and used by cells, and have discussed some, but by no means all, of the technologies used in the laboratory to analyse and manipulate DNA. However, in this final chapter a few of the uses of such technology will be considered, to give a flavour of the application of molecular genetics to the real world and perhaps suggest what developments lie in the future.

Biotechnology

In Chapter 11 we discussed the cloning of genes, and clearly the introduction of genes into new species is very important in the techniques of DNA manipulation. Thus, the techniques exist for the introduction of a gene into the genome of a new organism, and in theory that gene may be just about anything. However, simply placing a gene into the genome will not achieve any more than having that gene located in those cells. For the biotechnologist, the gene not only has to be put into the correct organism but it also has to be recognized and used by that organism. As an example, let us look at the use of **recombinant DNA technology** to produce a blood clotting factor. The biotechnologist has isolated the gene and placed it in a bacterial genome, and now needs to have the blood clotting factor produced by the bacteria, to enable the biotechnologist to isolate large amounts of the factor and ultimately make money. Therefore the gene has to be placed into the correct vector, using restriction endonucleases and ligation, and then the vector has to be introduced into the bacterial cells. But how do we ensure that the gene is expressed? Here are a few of the considerations that need to be made:

- The gene has to be full-length, including a start codon.
- The gene needs to be next to a promoter that will function in the host organism. This may not be the original promoter from the gene of interest. The strength of the promoter is important too. If a large amount of the product is needed then a strong promoter giving the right level of expression will be needed.
- The gene needs to be in the vector in the correct orientation. Don't forget that DNA is double-stranded and the sequences along the two strands are different. Only one strand will read the correct codon sequence.
- Where in the cell will the product be located? This consideration may be more important in eukaryotic expression systems. For example, the cellular location of proteins can be altered by the inclusion at the N-terminal end of the protein of a signal peptide. Proteins that are not normally secreted may be secreted if the correct gene sequences are included.
- What is the copy number of the vector? The higher the copy number the greater the levels of expression achieved.

Commonly, genes may be fused, or ligated, together before introduction into the vector, and the products will therefore be **fusion products**, as depicted in Figure 14.1. It may be that the fusion product is not needed, but fusion aided the expression or purification of the product. Subsequent cleavage and isolation of the protein may be required before use.

Having briefly discussed the technology, what is it being used for? To date, many recombinant proteins are being produced for a variety of reasons. Most biochemical catalogues will list **recombinant proteins** that can be used for research purposes, while others are being produced for medical reasons. A selection of these is listed in Table 14.1.

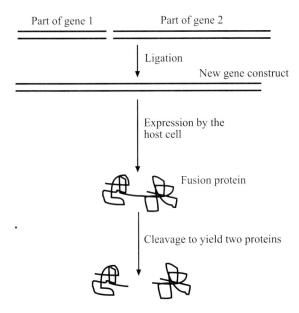

Part of gene 1   Part of gene 2

Ligation

New gene construct

Expression by the
host cell

Fusion protein

Cleavage to yield two proteins

Figure 14.1 *Production of fusion proteins from parts of two genes. The parts of the genes of interest are ligated together and expressed as one gene. The fusion product may be the product needed, but commonly it is cleaved to yield two proteins, only one of which may be required*

Biotechnology is also yielding other products using recombinant technology. Bacterial cells can be made to overproduce amino acids, or can be used to produce antibiotics. Microbes are also being used to produce polymers which have many uses in manufacturing or the food industry.

Many of the gene products are not simply native genes that are being expressed. As alluded to within the book, interest has been shown in how proteins such as *Taq* polymerase survive high temperatures. Once the secret to thermostability has been found, then it is sure to be engineered into many proteins which will be produced by recombinant technology. Meanwhile, the active sites of many enzymes are being studied.

Once it is known what makes up the active site of a protein and how it works, then alterations may be made. Alterations that may be required include:

Table 14.1 *Some proteins produced by biotechnology*

Product	Comment
Insulin	Used in diabetes
Tumour necrosis factor	Antitumour factor
Urokinase	Can be purified from urine
Interferons	Antitumour factors; promote white cell function
Interleukins	A growing list of cytokines
B-cell growth factor	Used in immune disorders
Antibodies	The specificity of these can be altered

The secret of thermal stability of proteins is important to biotechnologists because, if the temperature of a chemical reaction is raised by 10°C, then the rate of that reaction doubles. Therefore, raising the temperature of an enzyme producing an important product from 37°C to 80°C would substantially increase the rate of production of the desired chemical.

The active site of an enzyme is usually a small part which carries out the catalysis. The active site may be constructed from amino acids that are quite distant in the sequence, but which come together once the protein has been correctly folded. Once identified, such amino acids may be altered to change the functionality of the protein.

- Making the enzyme work faster.
- Allowing the enzyme to work under modified conditions, for example at a higher temperature or in a different solvent.
- Altering the substrates and/or products of the reaction catalysed by the enzyme.

One of the most widely used examples of protein engineering is the enzyme subtilisin in biological washing powder, where the enzyme was altered to enable it to function in the presence of detergents. It is hoped that in the future so much will be understood about protein folding and function that enzymes will be able to be designed from first principles and then the genes created and expressed to produce the perfect proteins for a particular function.

Transgenics

Transgenics is the incorporation of a gene from another source into the genome of an organism. The phrase is usually used in association with multicellular organisms. The gene to be incorporated is known as the **transgene** and it is usually incorporated and expressed with a resultant alteration of the phenotype of the host organism. Usually transgenics also refers to the fact that every cell of the organism contains the transgene, including the germ line cells, and therefore the transgene is passed on to successive generations. Commonly, the transmission of the transgene will follow the Mendelian inheritance patterns discussed in Chapter 8.

Plant transgenics

Plants have long been the target of transgenic technology and, by the development of better crop plants, not only do farmers potentially have greater profits but, more importantly, the world's food reserves can be increased to counter the ever growing population. Companies such as Monsanto and others have already launched genetically modified soya and tomatoes.

A few of the genetically engineered plants being sought are:

Companies such as Monsanto, who have already launched genetically modified products such as soya and tomatoes, are desperate to increase public awareness of the technologies they are using. Commonly, large advertisements are appearing in the popular media expressing the safety of such products.

- Herbicide-resistant plants. Crops are commonly sprayed with herbicides, but often crop damage will also take place. Manipulating the way in which the crop plants take up or metabolize the herbicide will potentially allow them to be resistant. Spraying to reduce weeds would then not affect the vital crop plants.

- Virus-resistant plants. Viruses can cause considerable damage to crops and by increasing their resistance to attack the crops can be protected. One approach is to express viral coat proteins in plants.

- Stress-tolerant plants. Plants are being sought that are resistant to heat, drought and UV damage. Often the damage involves oxygen free radicals, and by increasing the plant's levels of free radical scavenging enzymes some resistance can be conferred. Obviously, resistance to drought will be of great benefit in areas of the world where rainfall is uncertain.

- Insect-resistant plants. Insect damage to plants is a major problem. One approach is to attack the insects, but a second approach is to make the plants themselves resistant. Here work is already underway to introduce the production of insecticides such as protoxin into plants.

- Plant products with increased storage times. Millions of pounds of fruit and flowers are lost every year because of deterioration in storage or while being transported. By altering the ripening patterns and lengthening the stability of the plant products, the fruit, for example, could reach the consumer in a better condition and there would be less wastage.

- Plants as sources of biological materials. Under the correct conditions plants will grow quickly and quite rapidly a large amount of material can be harvested. Therefore, plants as bioreactors are seen as a feasible option. Antibodies and plastics such as polyhydroxybutyrate can be produced in plants. On a clinical note, vaccines can be produced in plants and then, to introduce the vaccine into humans, the fruits simply have to be eaten. Such ideas appear to have great potential.

Animal transgenics

Animals too are targets for transgenic technology. The transgene may be introduced by the use of a retrovirus, or alternatively **microinjected** in. The second of these two approaches is shown in Figure 14.2. Here, a fertilized egg is removed to culture, and the DNA construct containing the transgene is microinjected in while the egg still contains two **pronuclei**. By the incorporation within the construct of certain sequences, the transgene should become incorporated into the genome. Because the egg now has the transgene inside, and because this fertilized egg gives rise to all the cells of the organism, the final adult body should contain the transgene in every cell, including the germ line cells. Therefore, such an animal should be truly transgenic and be able to pass on the transgene to its offspring. However, as indicated in the figure (Figure 14.2), only a proportion of the animals born after the implantation of the manipulated eggs will be transgenic. There is a very high miss rate. The levels of expression of the transgene and the tissues in which the transgene is expressed are also important considerations. Often with mammalian transgenics, the transgene product should ideally be expressed into the milk, allowing easy isolation from the animal and easy further purification. Therefore the transgene construct employed in the first place has to use a promoter which is preferentially turned on in the lactating tissues,

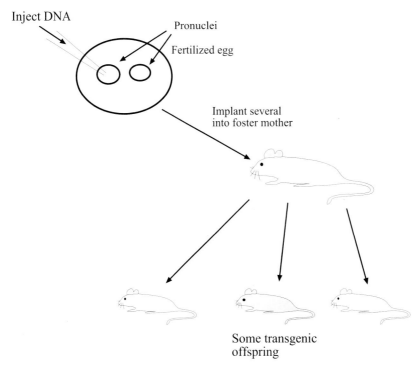

Figure 14.2   *One of the methods of producing transgenic animals. Here, the DNA is microinjected into the pronucleus of the fertilized egg and the modified eggs are transplanted into a foster mother. Not all the resulting animals will be transgenic*

Often microinjection into pronuclei is very difficult or impossible. Many fertilized eggs are opaque, making finding the pronuclei problematical. Often the transgene may be injected into the cytoplasm.

and the gene needs to have secretion sequences to ensure that the product is secreted into the milk.

A second way of obtaining transgenic animals is to use **embryonic stem cells** (ES cells). These are cells isolated from a developing **blastocyst** shortly after fertilization. The stem cells are cultured and the transgene construct added. The cultured cells can be selected and tested, perhaps with PCR, and enriched with respect to those cells in which the transgene has been incorporated. The resulting cells are then incorporated into a new blastocyst, which is subsequently implanted into a foster mother. However, as the new animal has arisen from cells that have been manipulated and cells from the second blastocyst, the resulting animal is a **chimera**. There is a chance that the germ cells carry the transgene and, if they do, then the animal can be bred from; but this is far from guaranteed.

What are the types of 'new' animals that are being created by this technology?

- Milk-producing animals as bioreactors, where recombinant proteins are produced in the milk.
- Animals producing better quality milk. The amounts of dairy products produced from the milk can be increased.

- Animals with a greater body mass. Here farm animals, or fish, may be bigger, yielding greater amounts of meat. Often meat quality is compromised.
- Fish which can survive lower temperatures via expression of an antifreeze protein.
- Animals which are resistant to viruses, bacteria and parasites.
- Mice as models of human diseases. By the use of antisense technology, for example, genes can effectively be stopped from being expressed, mimicking the situation where a gene is defective in a disease. The physiology of that animal may then be studied.

> Antisense technology enables the expression of a gene to be stopped. Here, a gene is placed in an organism which produces a RNA molecule which has the complementary strand to the RNA of the gene of interest. Hybridization of the RNA products of the two genes will then take place which will stop the translation of the genes into protein products. Therefore, although the gene of interest is still transcribed, effectively its expression has been stopped. This is often a technique used to study the role of gene products in cells.

Gene therapy

Although in transgenics the discussion concentrates on the incorporation of genes into plants and animals, humans too are potential targets for insertion of genes. Many human diseases are caused by defects in genes, and often single genes are known to be affected. Therefore, there is now the potential for the incorporation into the human genome of a correct version of the defective gene and, with the expression of such a gene in the right tissues at a high enough level, the disease can be corrected. Such an approach is termed **gene therapy**. At the moment, the only cells that are allowed to be manipulated are those of the non-germ line cells, the somatic cells. Therefore, the only gene therapy viable is **somatic gene therapy**, germ line gene therapy being forbidden.

> Gene therapy is defined as the delivery of a gene to an individual with the aim of permanently correcting a genetic disease caused by a defective version of that gene.

Some of the potential diseases which could be targets for gene therapy are listed in Table 14.2.

To date, little success has been achieved in gene therapy and some exponents claim that the technique will never work. However, large amounts of effort are currently being put into this area because of its potential power to permanently cure diseases. There are, however, many obstacles to overcome:

Table 14.2 *Potential diseases that are targets of somatic gene therapy, and the gene products needed to obtain a cure*

Disease	Gene product
Cystic fibrosis	Cystic fibrosis transmembrane regulator
Chronic granulomatous disease	NADPH oxidase components
Haemophilia B	Blood factor IX
Hypercholesterolaemia	LDL receptor
Duchenne muscular dystrophy	Dystrophin
Severe combined immunodeficiency (SCID)	Adenosine deaminase

- The gene has to be isolated. Commonly, this has now been done.
- The gene has to be introduced into the patient. This may be *in vivo*, where the gene construct is given directly to the patient, or *ex vivo*, where cells are removed from the patient, modified and then returned. Bone marrow may be a target here.
- The gene has to be expressed in the correct tissues.
- Integration of the gene and its expression need to be stable.
- Cost: gene therapy is very expensive to develop and use. With some diseases each patient is likely to be treated as an individual case. Many believe the cost is prohibitive.

Cloning

Although not in itself a new idea, in the mid-1990s came the announcement that a sheep had been cloned from an adult source of DNA. In this experiment, essentially a fertilized egg had all its DNA removed and then replaced with that from the nucleus of another cell. This 'new' egg was then implanted into a foster mother and a lamb was born. This lamb, named **Dolly**, was genetically identical to the original adult animal used as a source of DNA. The experiment had yielded many failures along the way but its final success meant that this was the first time that a mammal had been cloned from an adult, and the news of this success hit the world headlines. However, sceptics feared that the lamb would not be genetically the correct age. It is thought that, as cells age, then the DNA itself alters and, thus, taking this pre-aged DNA and putting it into a new egg to produce a new animal may mean that the DNA in the newborn is already the age of the parent animal. However, Dolly was able to become pregnant and had her own offspring, Polly.

In July 1998, the original researchers who created Dolly the sheep confirmed that she was cloned from adult cells as originally described, dispersing doubts that the sheep was not a true adult clone. On the same news bulletin was the announcement that a group in Hawaii had cloned a large group of mice from adult mice cells. The methods used appeared to be much improved over those used to create Dolly. Furthermore, the group had produced clones of the cloned animals, and it appears that cloning from adults is now going to be a viable technique in the near future.

Why would you need to clone mammals? As well as the fear that certain humans may wish to clone themselves, discussed briefly below, it is also of interest to the agricultural world. Once an individual animal is either bred or created by transgenics to be as good as possible at producing wool or meat, then cloning would allow a virtually unlimited and never-ending supply of such animals, without the need to repeat the long and difficult first steps.

Ethics and social considerations

The discussion of Dolly the sheep above leads us to the need to discuss the issue of ethics and the impact that this new technology is making on society. Many people fear that geneticists are 'playing at being God' and that they are 'interfering with nature'.

The cloning of Dolly hit the headlines all over the world and was even discussed in popular magazines. The fear was, or is, that certain rich or powerful individuals would wish to clone themselves and therefore continue. This, of course, is a misconstrued argument. Any new individual produced by cloning would not be the same individual as the donor of the DNA. Effectively one would be creating identical twins, but with an age difference of perhaps 30–50 years. These new babies would be individuals in their own right. However, the impact on a child later in life when their origin needs to be explained may be problematical. At the moment, cloning of humans is banned, but for how long? Cloning of animals is probably here to stay.

Cloning is not the only emotive issue. In August 1997, a failed attempt was made to destroy genetically modified crops in Devon, UK, which started a local protest against the growing of such crops. Farmers with nearby fields which had been classified as organic tried to take court action against the growing of the new crops and local MPs started to call for the South-west of England to become a genetically modified crop-free zone. Erroneous results by one scientist briefly added to the controversy, and clearly there is public concern about the growing of such plants in the open. It will be interesting to see how such protests develop, and how many of the new crops will appear in the supermarkets. There are fears that genetically modified food products might not be safe in the long term, and more research does need to take place in that area. Certainly, all food produced containing genetically modified material will have to be clearly labelled, and it will be interesting to see how soon the public accepts such products as being part of life.

Suggested further reading

Anderson, W.F. (1992). Human gene therapy. *Science,* **256,** 808–813.

Anderson, W.F. (1998). Human gene therapy. *Nature*, **392**, 25–30. (A more recent review.)

Cleaver, J.E. (1998). Hair today, gone tomorrow; transgenic mice with human repair deficient disease. *Cell*, **93**, 1099–1102. (Example of transgenics.)

Davies, J.C., Geddes, D.M. and Alton, E.W.F.W. (1998). Prospects for gene therapy for cystic fibrosis. *Molecular Medicine Today*, **4**, 292–299.

Flotte, T.R. and Carter, B.J. (1998). Adeno-associated virus vectors for gene therapy of cystic fibrosis. *Methods in Enzymology*, **292**, 717–732. (And other articles in this journal.)

Gasser, C.S. and Fraley, R.T. (1992). Transgenic crops. *Scientific American*, **266**, 62–69.

Glick, B.R. and Pasternak, J.J. (1994). *Molecular Biotechnology: Principles and Applications of Recombinant DNA*. ASM Press.

Gurdon, J.B., Laskey, R.A. and Reeves, O.R. (1975). The developmental capacity of nuclei transplanted from keratinized skin cells of adult frogs. *Journal of Embryology and Experimental Morphology*, **34**, 93–112. (Very early cloning experiments.)

Hughes, M.A. (1996). *Plant Molecular Genetics*. Longman (AWL).

Johnson, I.S. (1983). Human insulin from recombinant DNA technology. *Science*, **219**, 632–637.

Mulligan, R.C. (1993). The basic science of gene therapy. *Science*, **260**, 926–932.

Sudbery, P. (1998). *Human Molecular Genetics*. Longman (AWL). (Chapter on gene therapy in particular.)

Wakayama, T., Perry, A.C.F., Zuccotti, M., Johnson, K.R. and Yanagimachi, R. (1998). Full-term development of mice from enucleated oocytes injected with cumulus cell nuclei. *Nature*, **394**, 369–374. (Recent cloning of mice.)

Wells, J.A., Powers, D.B., Bott, R.R. *et al.* (1987). Protein engineering subtilisin. In *Protein Engineering* (Oxender, D.L. and Fox, C.F., eds.). ARL Inc.

Wilmut, I., Schieke, A.E., McWhir, J., Kind, A.J. and Campbell, K.H.S. (1997). Viable offspring derived from fetal and adult mammalian cells. *Nature*, **385**, 810–813. (First mammalian cloning: Dolly the sheep.)

Self-assessment questions

1. Why is Dolly the sheep significant to the world of genetics?
2. How do *in vivo* and *ex vivo* gene therapy differ?
3. If a gene is placed in a vector for expression in the host cell, why does the gene have to be in the correct orientation?
4. What is a fusion product?
5. List three recombinant proteins produced by the biotechnology industry.
6. What are the two main techniques used to introduce a transgene into an animal embryo to create a transgenic individual?
7. If a person uses their own DNA to clone themselves, have they recreated themselves?
8. How does germ line gene therapy differ from somatic gene therapy?
9. For a gene therapy cure of haemophilia B, which gene needs to be introduced into the patient?

Key Concepts and Facts

Biotechnology
- DNA technology can be put to a diverse range of uses, from the manufacture of biological compounds to the potential curing of diseases.
- To obtain the production of protein, the gene has to be expressed in the host cell.
- Many factors have to be considered to achieve successful gene expression in 'foreign' host cells.
- Fusion products are sometimes produced.

Transgenics
- Transgenics is the incorporation of a gene from one source into a new genome.
- The incorporated gene is known as the transgene.
- Plant products from transgenic technology are now used commercially.
- Plants can be produced that are resistant to herbicides, stress, viruses or insects.
- Transgenic animals can be created by microinjection of pro-nuclei, or by the use of embryonic stem cells.
- Animal transgenics can be used to produce better agricultural products or for models of disease.

Gene Therapy
- Several diseases are presently being targetted as being potentially curable by gene therapy, not least cystic fibrosis.
- Gene therapy is the introduction of a new gene into a patient, with the permanent correction of a genetic disease.
- Only somatic gene therapy is allowed at present.
- Introduction of the new gene can be carried out *in vivo* or *ex vivo*.
- Gene integration, successful expression and tissue specificity of expression need to be considered.

Cloning
- The cloning of animals using adult cells as a source of material is now possible.
- The first cloned mammal using adult DNA was Dolly the sheep.
- Cloning of adults could be used to perpetuate transgenic lines.

Ethics
- Cloning and genetic modification of crops are issues of public concern.
- Both debate and more research are needed before genetically modified products are widely accepted by the public.

Answers to self-assessment questions

Chapter 1

1. Gene therapy is the technology which allows the replacement of a defective gene in a person's genome.
2. Gregor Mendel, the monk, is the 'father' of modern genetics.
3. Hugo De Vries, Carl Corens and Erich von Tschermak rediscovered Mendel's work.
4. Alkaptonuria, in which a black pigment is secreted in the urine, was the first genetic disease characterized.
5. Morgan worked on *Drosophila melanogaster*.
6. George Beadle and Edward Tatum in 1941 proposed that one gene encoded for one enzyme.
7. The hypothesis should be 'one gene/one polypeptide'. This is because many enzymes are composed of more than one polypeptide, each of which requires its own gene.
8. James Watson and Francis Crick solved the structure of DNA.

Chapter 2

1. Because the sugar contains five carbon atoms, either as a linear chain or in a ring structure.
2. In DNA the pentose sugar is $2'$-deoxyribose. In RNA it is ribose. $2'$-Deoxyribose does not have an OH group attached to the carbon atom in the $2'$ position.
3. A nucleoside is a sugar attached to a base.
4. Pyrimidines = thymine and cytosine; purines = adenine and guanine.
5. A nucleotide is a nucleoside with phosphates attached to the $5'$ carbon of the sugar.
6. At one end there is still a triphosphate unit attached to the $5'$ carbon of the sugar, and therefore this end of the chain is called the $5'$ end. At the other end is an unused $3'$ carbon still attached to an untouched OH group. This is the $3'$ end of the chain.
7. X-ray diffraction. This technique is still regularly used to solve the structures of proteins.
8. Hydrogen bonding holds the strands of DNA together.

9. Thymine on one strand always hydrogen bonds to adenine on the other strand, while cytosine always hydrogen bonds to guanine.
10. A, B, C, D, E or Z are forms of the DNA helix.
11. Synthesis of new DNA is catalysed by DNA polymerase.
12. DNA synthesis always take place in the $5'–3'$ direction.

Chapter 3

1. No. Many genomes have large amounts of apparently redundant DNA.
2. In the $3'–5'$ direction.
3. A group of contiguous genes which are controlled in a co-ordinated way.
4. A non-functioning gene. One which does not encode a functional product or is not expressed.
5. Intervening sequences or, more commonly, introns.
6. Consensus sequences are sequences which are most likely to occur in related genes. Usually such sequences are found by the alignment of several related sequences, and the most likely nucleotides at each position would be quoted in the consensus sequence.

Chapter 4

1. A bacteriophage is a virus which uses bacteria as hosts.
2. An aliquot of the sample and bacteria would be spread on a solid medium and the presence of plaques in the bacterial lawn looked for after a period of incubation.
3. A single-stranded RNA between 6 kb and 9 kb.
4. Plasmids are small circular DNA molecules which exist independently in cells.
5. DNA is found in both mitochondria and chloroplasts.
6. A nucleosome is a structure comprising DNA and histone proteins. Nucleosomes associate together to form chromatin.
7. The ends of the chromosomes are called telomeres.
8. Mitochondrial genomes encode several very important proteins which are instrumental to the function of the organelle.

Chapter 5

1. Protein synthesis requires the processes of transcription and translation.
2. The sugar in RNA is ribose, not deoxyribose, and RNA utilizes the base uracil (U) instead of thymine (T).
3. The instability of mRNA enables the synthesis of proteins to be

controlled. If mRNA levels remained high in the cell, protein synthesis could continue unabated.

4. A poly(T) sequence can be used to preferentially hybridize to the poly(A) tail of mRNA.
5. tRNA is commonly depicted in a shape resembling a cloverleaf.
6. The amino acid attaches to the acceptor arm of a tRNA, where there lies a 5′-CCA-3′ sequence.
7. Prokaryotic ribosomes have a sedimentation coefficient of 70S, and consist of 50S and 30S subunits. Eukaryotic ribosomes are 80S and consist of 60S and 40S subunits.
8. The holoenzyme of RNA polymerase from *E. coli* has the subunit structure $\alpha_2\beta\beta'\sigma$.
9. Transcription takes place in the 3′ to 5′ direction.
10. Initiation of transcription takes place at the promoter.
11. Termination may be rho-dependent or rho-independent.

Chapter 6

1. RNA of the known sequence needed to be synthesized and translation in a cell-free system was needed.
2. UGUGU etc. would be read off as either UGU or GUG alternately. These two codons code for cysteine and valine and so the amino acid sequence would be Cys-Val-Cys-Val etc.
3. Colinearity means that the order of the bases in the DNA corresponds to the order of the amino acids in the protein.
4. A codon is a group of three consecutive bases which encode for an amino acid, or a stop signal.
5. The first amino acid incorporated is either methionine in eukaryotes or formyl-methionine in prokaryotes.
6. The three stop codons are UAA, UAG or UGA.
7. The double sieve hypothesis explains the selectivity of tRNAs.
8. Protein synthesis takes place in the N to C direction.
9. The factors involved in termination of translation are referred to as release factors.
10. A polysome is a length of mRNA associated with several ribosomes.
11. Inosine is a deaminated form of guanine.

Chapter 7

1. DNA/protein binding areas can be identified by carrying out a DNase protection experiment.
2. An operon is a set of contiguous genes with co-ordinated control.
3. It is polycistronic because it encodes more than one gene product.
4. The natural inducer of the lactose operon is allolactose formed by the action of β-galactosidase.

5. The second messenger is cAMP.
6. The C protein exerts both a positive and a negative regulation of the arabinose operon, whereas the repressor of the lactose operon only lowers the level of expression.
7. The nucleus.
8. Enhancers are sequences which are elsewhere on the DNA but have an influence on the promoter activity.
9. Structures found in transcription factors include: helix-turn-helix polypeptides, zinc fingers and leucine zippers.
10. Adenylate cyclase catalyses the formation of the second messenger cAMP.

Chapter 8

1. The F_2 generation would have a phenotype ratio of $3:1$.
2. Digenic inheritance patterns are usually represented as Punnett squares (see Table 8.2).
3. The common ratio for digenic inheritance is usually $9:3:3:1$.
4. The heterozygous plants are showing incomplete dominance.
5. The *MM* combination of alleles is fatal and the animals are stillborn.
6. Human females never inherit genes on the Y chromosome.
7. Individuals with Turner's syndrome lack one sex chromosome and are genotypically XO.
8. A frame-shift mutation is where the alterations in the bases, deletions or insertions, are not in multiples of three and therefore all subsequent codons are incorrectly read.
9. A nonsense mutation is when a stop codon is created, leading to a truncated gene product.

Chapter 9

1. Homologous recombination takes place between two sequences that are extensively the same.
2. Robin Holliday first suggested a mechanism for recombination and now we have the Holliday structure.
3. The units of a genetic map are map units or centimorgans (cM).
4. Gene transfer in bacteria may take place through conjugation, transduction or transformation.
5. The gene responsible for cystic fibrosis was found by chromosome walking.
6. Mendel stated that the segregation of alleles is independent of others, but clearly in mapping we rely on the fact that alleles are linked, physically, and thus independent separation of alleles is not possible in these cases.
7. The segment on a chromosome where a gene is said to reside is called its locus.

8. The F plasmid controls conjugation in bacteria.
9. Transduction is mediated by a phage in bacterial gene transfer.

Chapter 10

1. Southern analysis is used for DNA while Northern analysis is for RNA.
2. Western analysis is for the study of proteins.
3. Nitrocellulose is commonly used to bind to DNA.
4. The purity of RNA can be assessed by spectrophotometry or by gel electrophoresis.
5. DNA analysing gels are usually made using agarose, although polyacrylamide is also used sometimes.
6. Commonly, the probe is made radioactive and then its presence analysed by autoradiography.
7. The largest DNA fragments will be found nearest the top of the gel, while the smaller fragments will be nearest the bottom, having run the furthest.
8. Electrophoresis is the movement of charged molecules in an electric field.

Chapter 11

1. DNA may be isolated by phenol extraction or by ultracentrifugation. Alternative methods are also available.
2. Svedberg units (S) are those named after the Swede who developed the technique.
3. Density gradient centrifugation or velocity centrifugation may be used for DNA isolation.
4. DNA is cut by restriction endonucleases.
5. Ligases are used to join DNA together.
6. The white colonies are the ones you need to concentrate on, as these will have not only the vector but also the insert in the correct position within the vector.
7. Bacteriophages have an inherent method of getting the DNA into the cells, which plasmids don't.
8. A cosmid is a cross between a plasmid and a phage.
9. A cDNA library is a collection of vectors which contain cDNA fragments. These cDNA segments will be derived from RNA from the cell of interest, as opposed to fragments of the cell's original DNA (a genomic library).
10. The process of deriving a DNA sequence from an amino acid sequence is known as back-translation.
11. *Eco*RI was isolated from *E. coli*, the first three letters of the abbreviation indicating this.

Chapter 12

1. The specificity is dictated by the sequences of the specific primers that are used to target the desired product from PCR.
2. The three main steps in PCR are: (i) denaturing at 95°C; (ii) cooling for hybridization to approximately 54°C; (iii) reheating for DNA synthesis at 72°C.
3. DNA products from PCR are analysed by agarose gel electrophoresis.
4. DNA synthesis in PCR is usually catalysed by *Taq* polymerase. This is a polymerase from the thermophile *Thermus aquaticus*.
5. PCR primers are usually designed to be 200–6000 bases apart along the DNA.
6. Using PCR a researcher can ascertain whether the potential transgenic organism is indeed carrying the transgene and can also check it for correct integration into the genome.
7. RT-PCR stands for reverse transcriptase-polymerase chain reaction.
8. RT-PCR is used to find the presence of RNA. RNA is firstly copied to a DNA form, and then PCR used. Only if the RNA sequence was originally present will the sample contain a DNA copy and therefore amplification take place.
9. The polymerase chain reaction will double the DNA present with each cycle and therefore, after 20 cycles, we will have 2^{20} or 1 048 576 molecules present.
10. RAPD analysis can be used for comparisons of genomes.

Chapter 13

1. The Maxam–Gilbert method of DNA sequencing uses cleavage.
2. The Sanger dideoxy method relies on DNA synthesis termination.
3. A DNA sequencing autoradiograph is read from the bottom to the top (see Figures 13.2 and 13.3).
4. Nucleotides are fluorescently labelled for automated sequencing.
5. The open reading frame is the translated region between the start codon and the termination codon.
6. A double-stranded DNA can be translated six ways (see Figure 13.4).
7. SWISS-PROT is a protein sequence database.
8. Prosite is a database of consensus sequences.
9. Chou and Fasman devised a method of predicting protein structure.
10. The Human Genome Project hopes to completely map and sequence the human genome.

Chapter 14

1. Dolly was the first mammal to be cloned using an adult cell as the source of DNA.

2. *In vivo* means that the recombinant DNA was delivered directly to the patient. *Ex vivo* involves the removal of cells, the manipulation of those cells in culture and then their replacement back into the patient.

3. A double-stranded DNA has to be correctly orientated in an expression vector, as translation of the two strands will result in two different amino acid sequences, only one of which is correct.

4. A fusion product is a single polypeptide which is made from two genes that have been ligated together.

5. Recombinant proteins produced include, amongst many others: insulin; tumour necrosis factor; urokinase; interferons; interleukins; B-cell growth factor; and antibodies.

6. The transgene can be microinjected into the pronucleus of the fertilized egg or, alternatively, it might be introduced into embryonic stem cells which are subsequently introduced into a new blastocyst.

7. No. If an individual clones themselves, they merely create a new individual who is genetically identical – a situation little different to identical twins.

8. Germ line gene therapy means that the cells of the germ line have been manipulated and therefore changes are able to be passed on to the offspring. Somatic gene therapy is manipulation of non-germ line cells only.

9. To cure haemophilia B the gene needed is blood factor IX.

Index